SCOLIOSIS SURGERY FOR PATIENTS

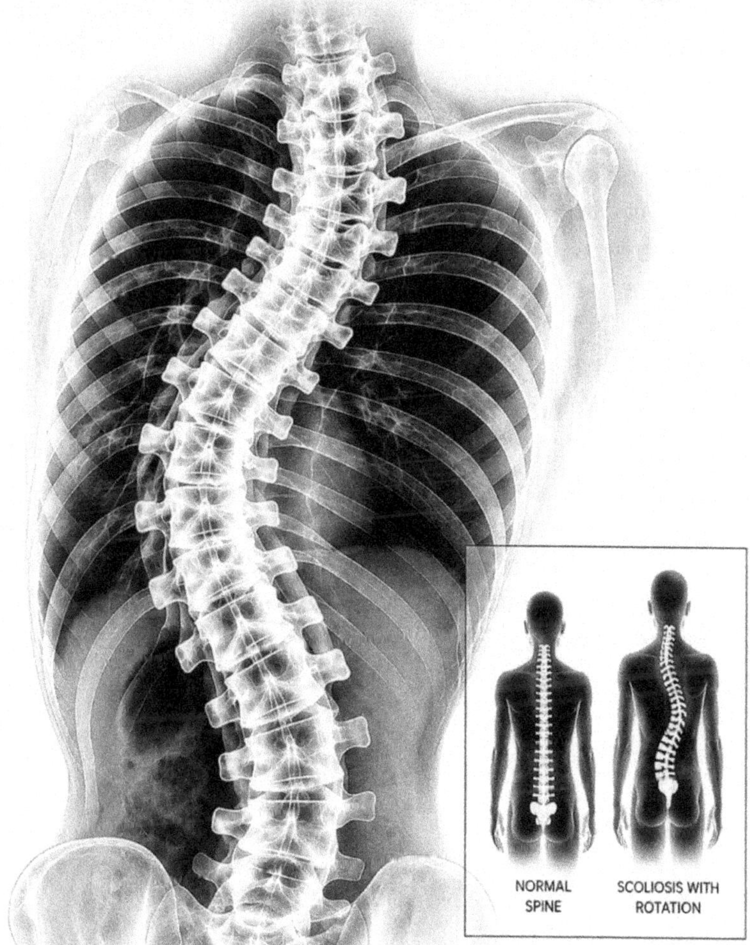

SAQIB A. SIDDIQUI, MD

Scoliosis Surgery for Patients

First Edition

ISBN (Paperback): 979-8-2561-7191-9
ISBN (Hardcover): 979-8-2561-7196-4
ISBN (eBook): 979-8-2561-7192-6

Published by:
USA Publishing Hub
Printed in the United States of America

TABLE OF CONTENT

Medical Disclaimer

This book is intended for educational purposes only. It is not a substitute for professional medical advice, diagnosis, or treatment. Always seek the guidance of your physician or qualified health provider with any questions you may have regarding a medical condition. Never disregard professional medical advice or delay in seeking it because of something you have read in this book.

The information contained in this book reflects the author's clinical experience and the published medical literature at the time of writing. Medical knowledge evolves, and specific recommendations may change over time.

AUTHOR'S NOTE

This book was written for one reason: because patients deserve to understand what is happening to their spine and why surgery, when recommended, is not something to fear but something to prepare for intelligently.

Over the course of my career as a spinal surgeon, I have sat across from hundreds of patients and their families in consultation rooms. I have seen the worry in their eyes. I have heard the same questions asked again and again, sometimes confidently, sometimes in a whisper. What exactly is scoliosis? Why does my curve need surgery when my friend's did not? What will my recovery look like? Will I be the same person afterward?

Those are not simple questions. They deserve complete answers, and that is what this book attempts to provide.

I want to be clear about what this book is and what it is not. It is an educational guide, a resource to help you understand the medical landscape of scoliosis surgery so that you can have better conversations with your own surgeon, make more informed decisions, and approach your journey with greater confidence. It is not a substitute for professional medical advice, and every patient's situation is unique. The information here reflects current best practices and the published literature, but your surgeon knows your specific anatomy, imaging, and health history in ways no book can replicate.

What I hope you take from these pages is not a checklist or a set of rules. I hope you take understanding. Because in my experience, the patients who do best, physically and emotionally, are the ones who arrive at surgery knowing what to expect and why it is necessary.

You are not just a patient. You are a person navigating one of the more significant decisions of your life. You deserve a guide that treats you that way.

I have organised this book to follow the natural sequence of the scoliosis surgical journey, from first understanding the condition through diagnosis, surgical decision-making, the operation itself, recovery, and finally the long-term picture of life after surgery. You do not need to read it from cover to cover, though you are welcome to. Each chapter is designed to stand on its own, so you can jump to the sections most relevant to where you are in your journey right now.

You will notice that each chapter ends with a section I have called From the Surgeon's Desk. These are personal reflections drawn from my clinical experience, the things I find myself saying again and again in consultation rooms, the observations that do not always fit neatly into a textbook but that matter enormously to real patients navigating real decisions. I hope these sections feel like a conversation rather than a lecture.

Throughout the text, medical terms are explained in plain language the first time they appear and are collected in a full glossary at the back. I have tried to write in a way that respects your intelligence without assuming a medical background.

This book is that guide. And you are exactly the reader it was written for.

How To Use This Book

This book is organised thematically, moving from foundational knowledge through to long-term outcomes. You do not need to read it cover to cover, though you are welcome to.

If you are newly diagnosed and trying to understand whether surgery is right for you, start with Parts One and Two. If you have already made the decision to proceed and want to prepare yourself practically and emotionally, focus on Parts Two and Three. If you are a caregiver supporting someone through this process, Part Three and the FAQ chapter will be especially practical. If you have already had surgery and are trying to understand what you are experiencing in recovery, Parts Four and Five are your most relevant sections.

Wherever you encounter a medical term in bold, it will be explained in plain language either immediately in the text or in the Glossary at the back of the book. Diagrams and illustrations are referenced throughout. Your surgeon can show you specific images related to your own case, and I encourage you to ask for that, because seeing your own spine on an image is one of the most powerful educational tools available.

At the end of most chapters, you will find a section called From the Surgeon's Desk. These are my personal reflections and clinical observations, the things I wish every patient knew before they came to see me, and the things I find myself repeating in consultation after consultation.

Take notes in the margins. Fold the pages. Bring this book to your appointments. Write your questions in the spaces provided. That is what it is here for.

One final note before we begin: this book will occasionally present statistical information and data from published research. When I cite figures, I have taken them from peer-reviewed studies and established clinical guidelines. Where evidence is uncertain or where practices vary between institutions and regions, I will say so. Medicine is not always a world of certainties, and I believe you deserve to know that honestly.

Now let us begin.

PART ONE

UNDERSTANDING SCOLIOSIS

CHAPTER ONE:

WHAT IS SCOLIOSIS? THE BASICS EVERY PATIENT SHOULD KNOW

Before we can talk about surgery, we need to talk about the spine itself. Not in the complicated language of a medical textbook, but in terms that make sense when you are sitting in a waiting room trying to understand what is happening to your body or your child's body. This chapter lays that foundation. Everything that follows in this book builds on what we cover here, so if you read nothing else carefully, read this.

THE REMARKABLE SPINE

The spine is one of the most extraordinary structures in the human body. It performs three critical functions simultaneously, and it performs them every moment of every day without you having to think about it. First, it provides structural support, holding the upper body upright against the constant downward pull of gravity. Second, it provides mobility, allowing you to bend, twist, reach, and move in nearly every direction. Third and perhaps most critically, it provides protection, encasing the spinal cord, the bundle of nerves that forms the communication highway between your brain and the rest of your body, in a bony tunnel that shields it from harm.

When the spine is working well, you barely notice it. It does its job in the background, silently and efficiently. When something goes wrong, it announces itself unmistakably. The spine's central role in virtually every movement the body makes means that spinal problems tend to have wide-ranging effects on daily life, which is exactly why conditions like scoliosis, when they progress, deserve serious attention and expert management.

To understand scoliosis, we need to first understand what a normal spine looks like, because the definition of scoliosis is essentially a deviation from that normal architecture.

WHAT A HEALTHY SPINE LOOKS LIKE

A healthy spine, when viewed from the side, has a series of natural, gentle curves. Looking at the neck region, the spine curves gently inward toward the front of the body. This is called the cervical lordosis. Moving down to the mid-back, the spine curves gently outward, away from the front of the body. This is called the thoracic kyphosis, and it is the curve responsible for the slight roundness of the upper back that is entirely normal and healthy. In the lower back, the spine curves inward again, creating the lumbar lordosis, which gives the lower back its characteristic gentle hollow.

These three curves work together like a precisely engineered spring. They absorb the vertical compressive forces generated by walking, running, and jumping, distribute load evenly across the vertebrae, and allow the upper body to maintain an upright position over the centre of gravity with minimal muscular effort. Remove any of these curves and the biomechanical efficiency of the spine is significantly compromised.

When you look at a healthy spine from the front or back, however, the picture is completely different. From this view, a normal spine appears as a straight vertical line. The individual vertebrae, the bones that make up the spine, are stacked directly on top of one another from the neck down to the pelvis, like a tower of blocks perfectly balanced on its base. There should be no deviation to the left or right.

Scoliosis disrupts this front-to-back symmetry. And it does so in a way that is more complex than it initially appears.

WHAT SCOLIOSIS ACTUALLY IS

The word scoliosis comes from the Greek word for crooked. In clinical medicine, scoliosis is formally defined as a lateral, meaning side-to-side, curvature of the spine measuring more than 10 degrees when measured on a standing X-ray using a standardised measurement system called the Cobb angle. We will explain the Cobb angle in detail shortly.

But here is the critical thing to understand about scoliosis that many patients are not told early enough: it is not simply a two-dimensional bend in the spine. In the vast majority of cases, scoliosis involves rotation of the vertebrae as well as lateral curvature. The vertebrae do not just tilt sideways, they also twist on their vertical axis.

Imagine a stack of building blocks that have each been shifted slightly to one side and also rotated a few degrees. If you view that stack from the front, you see the side-to-side curve. But the rotation adds an entirely different dimension of deformity, and it is this rotational component that creates many of the physical signs we associate with scoliosis: the rib hump that is visible when a person bends forward, the prominence of one shoulder blade, the asymmetry of the waist.

This three-dimensional nature of scoliosis is not just an anatomical curiosity. It has direct practical implications for how surgery is planned and executed. A surgical approach that simply bends the spine back toward straight without addressing the rotation would produce an incomplete correction. Modern scoliosis surgery addresses all three planes of the deformity simultaneously, which is one of the reasons why it is technically demanding and why the experience of the surgical team matters so much.

THE DIFFERENT TYPES OF SCOLIOSIS

Scoliosis is not a single condition. It is a description of a spinal finding, a lateral curve, that can arise from several entirely different underlying causes. Understanding which type of scoliosis a patient has is essential for treatment planning, prognosis, and surgical decision-making.

IDIOPATHIC SCOLIOSIS

The word idiopathic means of unknown cause, and idiopathic scoliosis is by far the most common type, accounting for approximately 80 percent of all scoliosis cases. In idiopathic scoliosis, the spine curves for reasons that despite decades of intensive research remain incompletely understood. Genetic factors appear to play a role, as scoliosis does run in families, but no single gene has been identified as the sole cause. Current research suggests that scoliosis likely arises from a combination of genetic predisposition, growth patterns, and biomechanical factors.

Idiopathic scoliosis is further classified by the age at which it develops, because age of onset has important implications for how the curve is likely to behave.

Infantile idiopathic scoliosis develops before the age of three. It is relatively uncommon and interestingly has different characteristics in different parts of the world, being more common in boys in Europe and more common in girls in North America. Many cases of infantile idiopathic scoliosis resolve spontaneously, but those that progress can become severe if not treated.

Juvenile idiopathic scoliosis develops between the ages of three and ten. This is a particularly important age group because these children still have significant skeletal growth remaining, which means curves can progress substantially if left untreated. Bracing and in some cases surgery are more frequently required in juvenile idiopathic scoliosis than in the infantile form.

Adolescent idiopathic scoliosis, often abbreviated to AIS, is the most common form, developing during the adolescent growth spurt between approximately 10 and 18 years of age. It affects girls more frequently than boys, with moderate to severe curves requiring treatment occurring approximately seven to eight times more often in girls. The reason for this sex difference is not fully understood. Adolescent idiopathic scoliosis is the form most likely to require surgical treatment when curves progress despite bracing.

Adult idiopathic scoliosis refers to curves in patients over 18 years of age. This category includes two distinct groups: patients who had adolescent scoliosis that was either undetected or not treated and have carried their curve into adulthood, and adults whose mild adolescent curves were stable for years but have begun to progress with age, often in association with disc degeneration and the biological changes of middle age.

DEGENERATIVE SCOLIOSIS

Degenerative scoliosis, also called de novo adult scoliosis or adult degenerative scoliosis, is a condition that develops in adulthood as a direct result of the wear and tear that affects the spine over time. It typically develops in patients over the age of 50, though it can appear earlier in patients with significant disc disease or other metabolic conditions affecting the spine.

The mechanism is relatively straightforward. As the intervertebral discs between the vertebral bodies lose height with age, and as the facet joints at the back of each vertebral level develop arthritis and degenerate unevenly, the vertebrae begin to tilt. When disc degeneration is asymmetric, occurring more severely on one side than the other, the vertebra above the degenerated disc tilts toward the side of greater collapse. This tilting is the beginning of the scoliotic curve.

Degenerative scoliosis predominantly affects the lumbar spine, the lower back. It is frequently accompanied by spinal stenosis, a narrowing of the spinal canal and the nerve exit foramina, which can cause significant leg pain, weakness, and difficulty walking. Managing this combination of deformity and neurological compression is one of the most complex challenges in adult spinal surgery.

CONGENITAL SCOLIOSIS

Congenital scoliosis arises from abnormalities in how the vertebrae formed during fetal development, typically during the first six weeks of pregnancy. These abnormalities can take several forms. A hemivertebra is a vertebra that formed incompletely, with bone present on only one side of the usual structure. Because a hemivertebra is essentially a wedge-shaped bone, it tilts the spine above it toward the side on which it is formed. A block vertebra occurs when two or more adjacent vertebrae fail to separate properly during development and remain fused together, creating a rigid segment that can cause progressive curvature at the levels above and below.

Because the structural abnormality is in the bones themselves rather than in the soft tissues and growth patterns, congenital scoliosis has a different natural history from idiopathic scoliosis and frequently requires earlier intervention. The management of congenital scoliosis requires a thorough understanding of the three-dimensional vertebral anatomy, often necessitating CT scanning and careful surgical planning.

NEUROMUSCULAR SCOLIOSIS

Neuromuscular scoliosis develops as a consequence of an underlying neurological or muscular condition. The list of conditions that can cause neuromuscular scoliosis is long, including cerebral palsy, muscular dystrophy in its various forms, spinal muscular atrophy, spina bifida, Friedreich's ataxia, and spinal cord injury among others. The common thread is that the muscles and nerves that normally maintain spinal alignment and support are weakened or unbalanced, allowing the spine to curve under the influence of gravity and uneven muscular forces.

Neuromuscular scoliosis tends to be more severe than idiopathic scoliosis, progresses more rapidly, and often produces curves that extend further, sometimes encompassing both the thoracic and lumbar spine and even the pelvis. Management of patients with neuromuscular scoliosis requires careful coordination between the spinal surgeon and the medical teams managing the underlying neurological or muscular condition, as well as detailed consideration of how the patient's underlying condition will affect surgical risk and recovery.

THE COBB ANGLE EXPLAINED

If you have had an X-ray for scoliosis, the term Cobb angle will almost certainly appear in the report, and your surgeon will use this measurement as a central part of their clinical decision-making. Understanding what it is and what it means will help you make sense of everything that follows.

The Cobb angle is the universally accepted standard measurement for quantifying the severity of a spinal curve. It was developed by Dr John Robert Cobb, an American orthopaedic surgeon, in the 1940s, and despite nearly eight decades of advances in spinal imaging and measurement technology, it remains the primary metric used to characterise scoliotic curves because of its simplicity, reproducibility, and the enormous body of clinical literature built on it.

To measure the Cobb angle, a standing full-length spinal X-ray is required. The radiologist or surgeon identifies the uppermost vertebra of the curve, called the upper end vertebra, and the lowermost vertebra of the curve, called the lower end vertebra. These are the vertebrae that are most tilted relative to the horizontal at the top and bottom of the curve. A line is drawn along the top surface of the upper end vertebra, and a line is drawn along the bottom surface of the lower end vertebra. The angle at which these two lines intersect, or would intersect if extended, is the Cobb angle.

The resulting measurement tells us the angular magnitude of the curve at the time of the X-ray. It is a snapshot, a moment-in-time measurement, which is why serial X-rays over time are so important in understanding whether a curve is stable or progressing.

Here is a practical guide to what Cobb angle measurements mean in clinical terms. A measurement of less than 10 degrees is not classified as scoliosis at all. It is considered normal variation in spinal alignment and does not require any specific management. Measurements between 10 and 24 degrees represent mild scoliosis. These curves are monitored with periodic clinical review and X-rays, and bracing may be considered in growing patients at higher risk of progression. Measurements between 25 and 44 degrees represent moderate scoliosis. In growing patients, bracing is typically recommended to prevent further progression. In adults, this range is monitored with ongoing observation and management of symptoms as they arise. Measurements of 45 degrees and above represent severe scoliosis, and it is in this range, with considerable nuance based on individual factors, that surgery is most commonly discussed.

It is essential to understand that the Cobb angle, while the universally used standard, is a two-dimensional measurement of what is fundamentally a three-dimensional problem. Two patients with identical Cobb angles can have very different clinical presentations, different levels of functional impact, different cosmetic concerns, and different surgical challenges depending on the location of the curve, the degree of rotation, the patient's overall spinal balance, and many other factors. This is why experienced scoliosis surgeons do not simply look at a number on a report. They look at the whole picture.

THE SIGNIFICANCE OF CURVE LOCATION

Not all scoliotic curves are equivalent even when they have the same Cobb angle measurement. The location of the curve within the spine has significant implications for its clinical impact, its risk of progression, and its surgical management.

Thoracic curves, those in the mid-back between T1 and T12, are particularly significant because the thoracic spine is surrounded by and attached to the rib cage. As a thoracic scoliotic curve progresses, the associated rotation of the vertebrae pushes the ribs on the convex side of the curve posteriorly and superiorly, creating the characteristic rib hump that is one of the most visible signs of thoracic scoliosis. In severe curves, this distortion of the rib cage can significantly reduce the space available for lung expansion, leading to reduced lung capacity and, in extreme cases, restrictive respiratory disease.

Lumbar curves, those in the lower back between L1 and L5, tend to cause different problems. They are often associated with significant pain because the lumbar spine bears the greatest load of the entire spinal column, and asymmetric loading across a curved lumbar spine accelerates disc degeneration. Lumbar curves also cause visible asymmetry of the waist and pelvis, with one hip appearing more prominent than the other.

Thoracolumbar curves span both the lower thoracic and upper lumbar regions. Double major curves describe a situation where there are two structurally significant curves, one in the thoracic and one in the lumbar spine, each curving in opposite directions. This pattern requires particularly careful evaluation because both curves must be assessed individually and in relation to each other when planning treatment.

THE DIFFERENCE BETWEEN A WATCHED CURVE AND A SURGICAL CURVE

One of the most common and completely understandable questions that patients and families ask is this: if my curve is 50 degrees and my friend's curve is also around that size, why does my surgeon recommend surgery but hers does not?

The answer is that the Cobb angle, while important, is only one of several factors that determine whether surgery is the appropriate recommendation. Others include the rate of progression, skeletal maturity, symptom burden, curve flexibility, the location and pattern of the curve, patient age, and the patient's own values and preferences.

A 50-degree curve in a 14-year-old girl who is still growing, whose curve has progressed 10 degrees in the past six months, and who is having difficulty with daily activities is a very different clinical picture from a 50-degree curve in a 35-year-old woman who has had essentially the same curve for 15 years with minimal symptoms and no evidence of progression. Both patients might well have surgery recommended, but the urgency, the rationale, and the surgical approach would be different.

Understanding this complexity is not meant to overwhelm you. It is meant to help you appreciate why the decision-making process requires an experienced specialist who knows your individual case, and why the conversation between you and your surgeon is so important.

FROM THE SURGEON'S DESK

One of the things that concerns me most when I meet new patients is that they have spent hours reading information online that is either outdated, overly frightening, or simply incorrect. The internet contains scoliosis forums where someone with a 15-degree curve shares the same space as someone preparing for a major spinal fusion, and the fear can bleed across cases where it does not belong.

So let me say this clearly: the vast majority of people with scoliosis will never need surgery. Most curves are mild, remain stable throughout life, and have no meaningful impact on longevity or overall quality of life. If you are reading this book, it is likely because surgery is at least being considered for your situation, which means your curve is more significant. But more significant does not mean hopeless, not even close.

Modern scoliosis surgery, performed by an experienced surgeon at a well-equipped centre with a dedicated team, achieves results that would have seemed extraordinary to surgeons even two or three decades ago. The correction rates are better. The safety profile is better. The recovery is faster. And the long-term outcomes, measured in decades of follow-up data from thousands of patients, are genuinely excellent.

The most important thing you can do right now is understand your specific situation. Know your Cobb angle and what it means. Know which type of scoliosis you have and how it tends to behave. Know what has been observed over time and what has changed. Know what the surgical recommendation is and why your surgeon is making it. The more you understand, the better partner you will be in your own care, and the better your outcome is likely to be.

Chapter Two:

The Spine — A Closer Look At Your Anatomy

You do not need a medical degree to understand spinal surgery. But you do need a working map of the territory. This chapter gives you that map, a clear and thorough guide to the anatomical structures that matter most when we talk about scoliosis, its effects, and its surgical correction. Take your time with this chapter. The knowledge you gain here will make every subsequent chapter clearer and more meaningful.

THE VERTEBRAE — THE BUILDING BLOCKS

The spine is made up of 33 individual bones called vertebrae. In adults, the bottom nine fuse together naturally during development, five forming the sacrum and four forming the coccyx or tailbone, leaving 24 mobile vertebrae that make up the functional spinal column.

These 24 mobile vertebrae are organised into three distinct regions, each with its own characteristic size, shape, and range of motion.

The cervical spine consists of seven vertebrae in the neck, labeled C1 through C7, counting from the top. The first two cervical vertebrae, C1 and C2, have unique shapes that allow for the specialised movements of the head. C1, called the atlas, is a ring-shaped bone with no vertebral body, designed to balance the skull. C2, called the axis, has a bony projection called the dens that fits up into the ring of C1, forming a pivot joint that allows the rotational movement of turning the head from side to side. The cervical spine as a whole has the greatest range of motion of any spinal region, which is why you can nod, shake, and tilt your head in so many directions. This mobility comes at the cost of vulnerability, as the cervical spine is also the region most susceptible to injury from trauma.

The thoracic spine consists of twelve vertebrae in the mid-back, labeled T1 through T12. Each thoracic vertebra articulates with a pair of ribs, one on each side, through specialized joints at the sides of the vertebral bodies and at the transverse processes (the bony projections on the sides). The rib cage formed by the thoracic vertebrae and the ribs attached to them creates a protective bony cage around the heart and lungs, provides attachment points for muscles of respiration and the upper limbs, and contributes significantly to the overall rigidity of the thoracic spine. This inherent rigidity means the thoracic spine has less range of motion than the cervical or lumbar spine, but it also means that thoracic scoliotic curves can be more rigid and harder to correct than curves in other regions.

The lumbar spine consists of five vertebrae in the lower back, labeled L1 through L5. These are the largest vertebrae in the spine because they must bear the greatest load. All the weight of the upper body, the head, arms, and trunk, is ultimately transferred through the lumbar vertebrae to the pelvis and then to the legs. The lumbar vertebrae have thick, broad vertebral bodies and large, sturdy bony processes. They allow good range of motion in forward and backward bending but are more restricted in rotation than the cervical spine.

THE ANATOMY OF AN INDIVIDUAL VERTEBRA

Each vertebra has a characteristic structure that is worth understanding in some detail, because the surgical techniques used in scoliosis surgery are directly related to the anatomy of the individual vertebral bones.

The vertebral body is the large, roughly cylindrical block of bone that makes up the front portion of each vertebra. It bears the main compressive load of the spine. The vertebral body consists of a shell of hard, dense cortical bone surrounding a core of softer, more porous cancellous bone. This structure gives it both strength and a degree of compressibility, allowing it to absorb some of the impact of normal activities.

Behind the vertebral body, a bony arch called the neural arch or vertebral arch encloses the spinal canal. This arch is formed by two pedicles, short stubby columns of bone that project backward from the sides of the vertebral body, which connect to two laminae, flat plates of bone that meet at the midline behind the spinal canal. The pedicles are of enormous surgical importance. They are the anchoring points for pedicle screws, the primary fixation device used in modern scoliosis surgery. Because the pedicle passes through the cortical shell of the posterior vertebral body, a screw placed through it and into the vertebral body can achieve very strong fixation in all directions.

Projecting from the neural arch are several bony processes. The spinous process projects directly backward from the junction of the two laminae. These are the bony bumps you can feel when you run your finger down the middle of your back. The transverse processes project sideways from the junction of the pedicle and lamina on each side. They serve as attachment points for muscles and ligaments. In the thoracic spine, they also articulate with the ribs. The articular processes project upward and downward from each vertebra and form the facet joints with the vertebrae above and below.

THE INTERVERTEBRAL DISCS

Between each pair of adjacent vertebral bodies sits an intervertebral disc. These discs are remarkable structures that serve several critical functions. They act as shock absorbers, cushioning the vertebrae from the impact of loading during walking, running, and all forms of movement. They serve as spacers, maintaining the height between adjacent vertebrae and thereby keeping the foramina, the exit channels for nerve roots, open and unobstructed. And they are flexible joints in their own right, allowing the limited bending and rotation between adjacent vertebrae that, summed across all disc levels, produces the considerable range of motion of the spine as a whole.

Each disc has two distinct components. The outer ring, called the annulus fibrosus, consists of multiple concentric layers of tough fibrocartilage arranged in a crisscross pattern. This arrangement, similar in principle to the layered structure of a car tyre, gives the annulus both tensile strength to resist being pulled apart and flexibility to allow controlled deformation under load. The inner core, called the nucleus pulposus, is a gel-like substance with a very high water content, particularly in young people. The nucleus pulposus acts as a hydraulic cushion, distributing compressive loads in all directions within the confines of the annulus.

As we age, the nucleus pulposus gradually loses its water content and becomes less gel-like and more fibrous. This is a normal part of aging, but it reduces the disc's shock-absorbing capacity and its ability to distribute load evenly. When disc degeneration is uneven, more severe on one side than the other, the result is asymmetric loading of the vertebrae, which is one of the primary mechanisms driving degenerative scoliosis in adults.

THE SPINAL CORD AND NERVE ROOTS

The spinal canal, the tunnel formed by the vertebral bodies at the front and the neural arches at the back, contains the spinal cord and the nerves that branch from it. Understanding the layout of these neurological structures is essential for understanding why protection of the nervous system is the paramount concern in scoliosis surgery.

The spinal cord is the direct continuation of the brain stem downward through the spinal canal. It carries all the nerve signals that travel between the brain and the body. Motor signals, the commands from the brain to the muscles that direct movement, travel down the spinal cord in specific tracts. Sensory signals, the information from the body about touch, temperature, pain, and position, travel up the spinal cord in different tracts. This functional separation means that different types of neurological injury can affect movement and sensation in different ways.

In adults, the spinal cord itself ends at approximately the L1 or L2 vertebral level. Below this, the spinal canal contains the cauda equina, a Latin term meaning horse's tail, referring to the bundle of nerve roots that supply the lower limbs, the bladder, the bowel, and the genitals. These individual nerve roots descend from the end of the spinal cord through the lower lumbar spinal canal to exit at their respective levels.

At each spinal level, paired nerve roots exit the spinal canal through the intervertebral foramina. There are two foramina at each level, one on the left and one on the right, each formed by the notches in the pedicles of the vertebrae above and below, and bounded by the disc at the front and the facet joint at the back. These nerve roots, once outside the spinal canal, form the peripheral nerves that supply specific regions of the body with motor and sensory function.

In scoliosis surgery, there are two primary neurological concerns. The first is the risk of injury to the spinal cord itself, which could cause weakness or paralysis of the legs, as well as loss of bladder and bowel control. This risk is managed through intraoperative neurophysiological monitoring, which we will discuss in detail in the surgical chapters. The second is the risk of injury to individual nerve roots as screws are placed near them or as the spine is moved during correction, which could cause pain, numbness, or weakness in the specific region of the body that nerve root supplies.

THE FACET JOINTS AND SPINAL STABILITY

The facet joints, also called zygapophyseal joints or Z joints, are the small paired joints at the back of each vertebral level. Each facet joint is formed by the inferior articular process of the vertebra above articulating with the superior articular process of the vertebra below. Like all synovial joints, facet joints have cartilaginous surfaces and are enclosed within a capsule containing synovial fluid.

The orientation of the facet joints varies in different regions of the spine and directly influences the directions of movement each region allows. Lumbar facet joints are oriented in a way that allows good flexion and extension but restricts rotation, which is why twisting movements in the lower back can be more stressful and injury-prone. Thoracic facet joints are oriented to allow more rotation, contributing to the rotational component of thoracic scoliosis.

As the spine degenerates, facet joint arthritis is one of the primary contributors to chronic back pain in adults. Arthritic facet joints develop bony spurs, called osteophytes, that can encroach on the spinal canal or the foramina, contributing to stenosis and nerve compression.

THE MUSCLES OF THE BACK

The spine does not hold itself upright. A sophisticated network of muscles provides the dynamic support that maintains spinal alignment during movement and resists the forces of gravity that constantly act on the spine.

The paraspinal muscles are the large muscles that run along either side of the spine from the pelvis to the skull. They are the primary movers of the back in bending and extending, and they play a crucial role in maintaining upright posture. In scoliosis, these muscles are asymmetrically loaded because the curved spine places them under uneven tension. Over time, this can lead to asymmetric muscle development, with the muscles on the concave side of the curve working harder and potentially becoming tighter and shorter than those on the convex side.

Deeper to the paraspinal muscles lies a series of shorter muscles that connect adjacent vertebrae or span just a few vertebral levels. The multifidus, one of the most important of these, runs from the sacrum up through the lumbar and thoracic spine. Research has shown that the multifidus is critical for spinal stability and that it is one of the muscles most affected by spinal surgery, both in terms of the disruption of the operation itself and in the post-operative recovery of spinal stability.

THE LIGAMENTS OF THE SPINE

Ligaments are tough, fibrous connective tissue structures that connect bones to other bones and provide passive stability to joints. The spine has several important ligament systems.

The anterior longitudinal ligament runs down the front of all the vertebral bodies and discs from the skull to the sacrum. It is a broad, strong band that resists extension (backward bending) of the spine and helps prevent excessive separation of the vertebral bodies at the front. The posterior longitudinal ligament runs down the back surface of the vertebral bodies within the spinal canal. It is narrower than the anterior longitudinal ligament and provides some resistance to flexion as well as helping to contain disc material in the spinal canal.

The ligamentum flavum is a paired ligament that connects the laminae of adjacent vertebrae, forming part of the back wall of the spinal canal. It is distinctive for its high content of elastic fibers, which give it a yellowish colour and allow it to stretch during spinal flexion and then return to its resting length on extension. In spinal stenosis, the ligamentum flavum can become thickened and buckle into the spinal canal during extension, contributing to nerve compression.

SPINAL BALANCE

One concept that surgeons think about constantly, and that patients often hear mentioned but rarely have properly explained to them, is spinal balance. A spine that is structurally aligned and mechanically efficient is described as being in balance, and restoring and maintaining spinal balance is one of the primary goals of scoliosis surgery.

Coronal balance refers to the alignment of the spine in the front-to-back X-ray view. In a well-balanced spine in the coronal plane, a vertical line drawn from the centre of the seventh cervical vertebra (C7) should pass through the centre of the sacrum. If this line falls to one side of the sacrum, the trunk is shifted to that side, creating asymmetric loading and visible postural imbalance.

Sagittal balance refers to the alignment of the spine as seen from the side. In a well-balanced spine in the sagittal plane, the natural cervical lordosis, thoracic kyphosis, and lumbar lordosis work together to position the body's centre of gravity over a stable base. When sagittal balance is disrupted, for example when the lumbar lordosis is reduced or reversed by degenerative changes or by fusion in an unfavourable position, the patient must work much harder to maintain upright posture, using muscle energy that a balanced spine would not require. Poor sagittal balance is strongly associated with chronic pain, functional limitation, and poor quality of life.

In planning scoliosis surgery, achieving good coronal and sagittal balance is not merely an aesthetic goal. It is a functional imperative that directly determines how well the patient will feel and function in the years and decades after surgery.

FROM THE SURGEON'S DESK

Patients sometimes look slightly surprised when I spend time on anatomy before we discuss the operation. They came to hear about surgery, not a biology lesson.

But here is the thing: patients who understand their own anatomy ask better questions, feel less anxious in the operating room, and recover with a clearer sense of what their body is doing and why. When I tell a patient post-operatively that instrumentation extends from T4 to L2, I want them to understand what that means, which vertebrae are involved, and why those levels were chosen. When I tell them that their sagittal balance has been significantly improved, I want them to appreciate the functional significance of that achievement.

The spine is not a mystery. It is an extraordinary, understandable structure, and knowing it is one of the most empowering things you can do as a patient navigating this process. Take the time to learn it well.

CHAPTER THREE:

DIAGNOSING SCOLIOSIS THE JOURNEY TO SURGERY

For most patients, the path to a scoliosis surgery consultation is rarely a straight line. It begins with an observation, sometimes a parent's worried glance at their child's uneven shoulders, sometimes a school nurse flagging an asymmetric posture during a routine check, sometimes an adult gradually developing back pain that does not respond to the usual treatments and finally prompts an imaging study that reveals a curve that has been there for years. From that first observation to a meaningful decision about surgery, there is almost always a period of investigation, monitoring, and careful consideration that can span months or years. This chapter walks you through that entire diagnostic journey.

HOW SCOLIOSIS IS FIRST DETECTED

In children and adolescents, scoliosis is most commonly first detected through three pathways.

School screening programmes are widely implemented in many countries as a means of detecting scoliosis early, when curves are smaller and more amenable to conservative management. During these screenings, a health professional typically performs the Adam's Forward Bend Test on every student. This is a simple examination that takes less than a minute but can detect spinal asymmetry with reasonable sensitivity.

Routine paediatric health checks with a family doctor or paediatrician are another common detection pathway. Alert clinicians who examine children regularly can identify early signs of scoliosis during routine well-child visits, particularly if they have a concern about posture or if a parent has mentioned observing asymmetry.

Parental observation is frequently the first step. Parents who notice that their child's clothes are fitting asymmetrically, that one shoulder appears higher than the other, that one hip seems more prominent, or that there is an unusual bulge on one side of the back when the child bends forward should seek medical evaluation. These observations should always be taken seriously.

In adults, scoliosis is often detected when imaging is performed for another reason, most commonly back pain. A GP refers a patient for an X-ray to investigate lumbar back pain, and the radiologist's report mentions a scoliotic curve that may have been present for years without causing specific symptoms, or may represent a degenerative curve that has developed more recently.

THE ADAM'S FORWARD BEND TEST IN DETAIL

The Adam's Forward Bend Test remains the most widely used clinical screening tool for scoliosis because it is simple, quick, requires no equipment, and can be performed by any trained health professional. It specifically assesses the rotational component of scoliosis rather than just the lateral curve, making it more sensitive than simple visual inspection in standing.

To perform the test, the patient is asked to stand with feet together, then bend forward slowly at the waist, keeping knees straight and arms hanging loosely with palms together, as though they are about to dive into a pool. The examiner observes the back from behind, and specifically from a position at the level of the back, looking down the length of the spine.

What the examiner looks for is asymmetry in the height of the ribs or the lumbar musculature on the two sides. In a patient with thoracic scoliosis, the rotational component of the deformity pushes the ribs on the convex side of the curve posteriorly and superiorly during forward flexion, creating a visible rib hump on that side. In lumbar scoliosis, a similar rotational asymmetry creates prominence in the lumbar paraspinal muscles on one side.

A scoliometer is a small inclinometer device that can be placed across the back during the forward bend to measure the angle of trunk rotation quantitatively. An angle of trunk rotation above 5-7 degrees is generally considered significant enough to warrant X-ray evaluation.

It is important to understand that the Adam's Forward Bend Test is a screening tool, not a diagnostic one. A positive test should always prompt further investigation with standing X-rays. A negative test does not completely exclude scoliosis, particularly for curves in the thoracolumbar region where the rotational component may be less pronounced.

IMAGING STUDIES — THE FOUNDATION OF DIAGNOSIS

Once scoliosis is clinically suspected, imaging is essential both to confirm the diagnosis and to characterize the curve fully so that appropriate management decisions can be made.

Standing Full-Length Spinal X-Rays

The cornerstone of scoliosis assessment is the standing full-length spinal X-ray. These are X-rays that capture the entire spine, from the base of the skull to the top of the sacrum, on a single image, taken in both the front-to-back view, called the anteroposterior or AP view, and the side view, called the lateral view.

The requirement that these X-rays be taken standing is critically important and is worth explaining. When a patient lies down, gravity no longer acts along the axis of the spine, and the compressive and shear forces that influence spinal alignment in everyday life are removed. A supine X-ray of a patient with significant scoliosis will show a smaller curve than the same patient's standing X-ray, sometimes dramatically so. Since we are interested in how the spine actually functions during daily life, standing X-rays are the only appropriate study for assessing scoliosis severity.

From standing full-length X-rays, the treating surgeon can measure the Cobb angle of each significant curve, determine the level of the end vertebrae, assess the degree of vertebral rotation, evaluate coronal and sagittal balance, determine the skeletal maturity of the patient using the Risser sign, identify any associated structural abnormalities, and monitor curve progression over time by comparing serial studies.

FLEXIBILITY STUDIES

Before surgical planning, most surgeons order flexibility X-rays in addition to standard standing views. These are X-rays taken while the patient bends maximally to the right and to the left, sometimes supplemented by traction views in which a gentle longitudinal force is applied to the spine while the X-ray is taken.

The purpose of flexibility studies is to assess how much of the curve is structural, meaning rigid and unlikely to correct spontaneously, versus how much is compensatory or flexible, meaning due to positional factors that will resolve when the structural curve is corrected. A curve that corrects substantially on a bending view is more likely to be fully correctable with surgery than a rigid curve that shows little change.

Understanding curve flexibility also guides decisions about which levels need to be included in a fusion. If an adjacent compensatory curve corrects fully on bending views, it may not need to be fused, which is desirable because every level preserved from fusion maintains useful spinal motion.

MAGNETIC RESONANCE IMAGING

MRI (Magnetic Resonance Imaging) uses powerful magnetic fields and radio waves rather than X-ray radiation to create detailed images of the soft tissues of the spine. It provides exquisite visualisation of the spinal cord and nerve roots, the intervertebral discs, and the ligaments, information that plain X-rays cannot provide.

MRI is not routinely required for the initial assessment of straightforward adolescent idiopathic scoliosis, because in this common condition the risk of associated intraspinal pathology is low. However, MRI is essential or strongly indicated in a number of specific situations. Atypical curve patterns, particularly left-sided thoracic curves, which curve in the opposite direction to the usual right thoracic pattern of adolescent idiopathic scoliosis, significantly raise the suspicion of an underlying spinal cord abnormality such as a syringomyelia, which is a fluid-filled cavity within the spinal cord, or a Chiari malformation, which is a condition in which brain tissue extends into the spinal canal. Neurological symptoms at any age, including weakness, numbness, tingling, or bowel and bladder dysfunction, mandate MRI evaluation. Rapid curve progression in a young patient and any suspicion of an underlying spinal cord tethering or other intraspinal abnormality also warrant MRI.

In adult patients, MRI is almost always performed as part of surgical planning, because disc degeneration, nerve root compression, and associated soft tissue changes are almost universally present and must be fully understood before surgery is undertaken.

CT SCANNING

Computed tomography, or CT scanning, uses X-rays acquired from multiple angles and processed by computer to create detailed three-dimensional images of the bony anatomy. While it involves higher radiation exposure than plain X-rays and does not show soft tissues as well as MRI, it is invaluable in specific circumstances.

In congenital scoliosis, CT scanning is essential to map the three-dimensional anatomy of malformed vertebrae before surgical planning. In patients with previous spinal surgery where implants may create artefact on MRI, CT provides the clearest images of the bony anatomy. In cases of severe and rigid deformity where the relationships between vertebrae are complex and difficult to understand from plain X-rays, three-dimensional CT reconstruction gives the surgeon a virtual model of the deformity from any angle.

Modern CT scanning technology, combined with surgical planning software, now allows surgeons to simulate the correction they plan to achieve before ever entering the operating room, which significantly improves surgical precision and reduces intraoperative surprises.

ASSESSING SKELETAL MATURITY WHY IT MATTERS

In growing patients, one of the most important clinical assessments is skeletal maturity, an evaluation of how much of the patient's growth potential remains. This matters enormously because curves in growing patients carry a much higher risk of progression than curves in patients whose growth is complete, and the amount of growth remaining directly influences treatment decisions.

The Risser sign is the most widely used measure of skeletal maturity in the context of scoliosis assessment. It is visible on the standard standing spinal X-ray and requires no additional imaging. The Risser sign refers to the ossification of the iliac apophysis, a crescent-shaped growth plate along the top of the iliac crest, the upper rim of the pelvis. Bone formation progresses from the front to the back of this growth plate as skeletal maturity advances. The Risser sign is graded from 0, meaning no ossification has appeared, indicating significant growth remaining, to 5, meaning the apophysis has fully fused with the iliac crest, indicating skeletal maturity.

A patient with a Risser sign of 0 and a 35-degree curve has a very different prognosis from a patient with a Risser sign of 4 and the same curve. The first patient is at high risk of significant curve progression during the remaining growth period. The second patient is near the end of growth and carries a much lower risk of progression.

Bone age assessment using a left hand and wrist X-ray provides complementary information. The growth plates of the bones of the hand close in a predictable sequence as skeletal maturity advances. Comparing the appearance of these growth plates to standards established from population studies allows estimation of the patient's biological age, which may differ from their chronological age and which can provide useful additional information in borderline cases.

Peak height velocity, the period of maximum linear growth during adolescence, is the period of greatest risk for curve progression. Clinical assessment of whether a patient has entered, is at, or has passed peak height velocity is an important clinical judgment that experienced surgeons incorporate into their risk assessment.

THE IMPORTANCE OF SERIAL MONITORING

Scoliosis is not a static condition, particularly in growing patients. Curves that are observed rather than treated require regular clinical review and periodic imaging to detect progression before it reaches a threshold requiring intervention.

Typical monitoring intervals for mild to moderate scoliosis in a growing patient are every four to six months during periods of active growth, with the interval extended to annually or as needed once growth is complete. Each visit includes clinical assessment and, at intervals determined by the clinical picture, a standing full-length spinal X-ray.

The practical implication of this monitoring programme is that patients and families must maintain regular engagement with their medical team over what can be a period of several years. Missing scheduled appointments can mean that curve progression goes undetected until it has advanced beyond the window in which less invasive treatments remain appropriate.

FROM THE SURGEON'S DESK

One of the most important moments in any consultation is when I show a patient their own X-ray for the first time. Some patients have been told they have scoliosis for years without ever actually seeing their spine. They know the word, they may even know their Cobb angle number, but they have never seen the image.

I always take time to walk through the film in detail. Here is your curve. Here is where it begins and ends. Here is the rotation we are seeing, and here is why the right side of your rib cage sits differently to the left. Here is where you are in terms of growth. Here is how the picture compares to where you were six months ago.

When patients see it, something changes. It becomes real, concrete, understandable. The abstract medical problem becomes their specific, visualisable situation, and that makes everything that comes next easier to engage with.

I also always emphasise that the imaging tells us the structure of the problem, but the clinical examination tells us the person. A severe curve in a patient who is asymptomatic, fully active, and unconcerned about appearance is a completely different consultation from a moderate curve in someone who is in daily pain and whose quality of life is significantly affected. The numbers matter. But the person in front of me matters more.

CHAPTER FOUR:

WHEN IS SURGERY RECOMMENDED? UNDERSTANDING THE INDICATIONS

This is the question at the heart of most consultations: why does this specific curve, in this specific person, need an operation? It is a fair question, and it deserves a thorough and honest answer. Surgery for scoliosis is not recommended lightly. It is a major undertaking for the patient, the family, and the surgical team. The decision to recommend surgery is made when the weight of evidence clearly shows that the benefits of surgical correction outweigh the risks of proceeding, and when the risks and consequences of leaving the curve untreated outweigh the risks of the operation itself.

Understanding the reasoning behind this decision will not only help you engage more meaningfully with your surgeon but will also give you confidence that the recommendation you have received is grounded in solid clinical evidence.

THE NATURAL HISTORY OF SCOLIOSIS WHAT HAPPENS WITHOUT TREATMENT

Before we can properly understand surgical indications, we need to understand what the evidence tells us about what happens to scoliotic curves when they are not treated. This is what clinicians call the natural history of the condition, and it is the essential reference point against which the risks and benefits of any treatment must be measured.

For mild scoliosis, meaning curves below 30 degrees in patients who have completed skeletal growth, the evidence is reassuring. Studies following these patients for decades have found that most mild curves remain essentially stable throughout adult life, with less than

10 degrees of additional progression on average. These patients generally experience no greater back pain or functional limitation than the general population, and their life expectancy is normal.

For moderate scoliosis in growing patients, meaning curves between 25 and 45 degrees in adolescents who still have significant growth remaining, the picture is more complex. These curves carry a real and significant risk of progression during the remaining growth period. Studies have shown that a moderate curve combined with young age and low Risser sign is associated with a greater than 60 percent probability of curve progression of 10 degrees or more during the remaining growth period. The faster the child is growing and the more growth that remains, the higher the risk.

For larger curves, the natural history becomes more concerning. Curves above 50 degrees at skeletal maturity are at significant risk of continued progression throughout adult life, often at a rate of approximately one degree per year, though this is highly variable. Over decades, this progressive worsening can lead to severe deformity, significant back pain, and in the case of thoracic curves, progressive reduction in lung capacity.

Large thoracic curves, particularly those exceeding 70 to 80 degrees, can cause clinically significant restrictive lung disease by distorting the rib cage and reducing the space available for lung expansion. In historical series from the era before effective surgical treatment, patients with severe untreated thoracic scoliosis had shortened life expectancy due to cardiorespiratory complications. Modern surgical treatment effectively prevents the development of this severe degree of pulmonary compromise.

THE GENERAL SURGICAL THRESHOLD AND WHY 45 TO 50 DEGREES IS SIGNIFICANT

In adolescent idiopathic scoliosis, the most widely cited surgical threshold is a Cobb angle of 45 to 50 degrees or greater in a growing patient, or above 50 degrees in a skeletally mature patient. This threshold is not an arbitrary number. It reflects the intersection of two curves on the natural history graph: below this threshold, the risk of significant long-term progression in adult life is relatively low, and the balance of risk does not clearly favour major surgery. Above this threshold, the risk of long-term progression, functional decline, and in severe cases cardiopulmonary compromise becomes substantial, and the evidence supports that the benefits of surgical correction reliably outweigh the risks of the procedure.

This threshold also reflects practical surgical realities. Curves below 45 degrees are generally more flexible and more fully correctable than larger curves. Performing surgery at a stage before significant curve rigidity has developed gives better surgical outcomes in terms of correction achieved. Waiting until a curve has progressed well beyond 50 degrees may result in a more technically challenging operation with less complete correction.

However, it is critical to emphasise that these are general guidelines, not rigid rules. Every patient's situation is evaluated individually, and the actual decision to recommend surgery takes into account many factors beyond just the Cobb angle.

CURVE PROGRESSION AS AN INDEPENDENT INDICATION

Even in a patient who has not yet reached the 45 to 50 degree threshold, surgery may be recommended if the curve is progressing rapidly. Progressive curves present a different risk profile from stable curves of similar size, because the trajectory they are on will, if unchecked, carry them through the surgical threshold and beyond.

In clinical practice, a curve that has increased by 5 or more degrees over a 3 to 6 month period in a growing patient is considered progressive and warrants escalation of management. If bracing has been attempted and the curve has continued to progress despite good brace compliance, surgery becomes the appropriate next step. This represents not a failure of the patient or the brace, but a recognition that the biological forces driving progression in that particular patient are stronger than what bracing can resist.

Documenting progression requires at least two measurements taken at different time points, ideally using the same projection and measurement technique to minimise measurement variability. A single measurement, no matter how high the Cobb angle, cannot tell us about trajectory. Two measurements over time can.

THE IMPACT OF SKELETAL MATURITY ON SURGICAL TIMING

Skeletal maturity is perhaps the most important modifier of surgical decision-making in adolescent scoliosis. A growing patient has two compelling reasons to consider earlier intervention compared to a skeletally mature patient: they are at higher risk of curve progression, and their more flexible curves are more completely correctable.

A 40-degree curve in a 12-year-old girl with a Risser sign of 0 who is growing rapidly is treated with significantly more urgency than the same curve in a 16-year-old with a Risser sign of 3 who has nearly completed growth. In the first patient, without intervention, that curve is very likely to progress to surgical thresholds and beyond during the remaining years of growth. In the second patient, the risk of significant further progression is considerably lower.

This is why timing matters in scoliosis management. Bracing is most effective during active growth, when the bone is most responsive to the compressive forces the brace applies. Surgery, when indicated, achieves better correction in more flexible curves, which are more likely to be encountered earlier in the disease course. Delaying surgical intervention unnecessarily in a rapidly progressing curve in a growing patient means potentially operating on a larger, more rigid, more complex deformity later.

NEUROLOGICAL SYMPTOMS AS AN URGENT INDICATION

Any scoliotic curve associated with neurological symptoms demands urgent investigation and may require prompt surgical intervention. Neurological symptoms in the context of scoliosis include weakness of the legs, numbness or tingling anywhere below the level of the curve, difficulty with gait or balance, and any loss of bladder or bowel control.

These symptoms suggest that the deformity or an associated intracanalicular abnormality is compromising the function of the spinal cord or nerve roots. Detailed neurological assessment and urgent MRI imaging are indicated whenever these symptoms are present. If a structural cause of neurological compromise is identified, surgery to address it should not be delayed.

THE ROLE OF PAIN AND QUALITY OF LIFE

For adults with scoliosis, the indication for surgery is more frequently driven by symptoms than by curve size alone. An adult with a 45-degree lumbar curve that has been stable for twenty years may have little reason for surgical intervention if they are asymptomatic or have only mild, manageable pain. The same curve in a patient who has progressively worsening pain, difficulty walking, neurogenic claudication, significant functional limitation, and markedly reduced quality of life presents a compelling case for surgical consideration.

The threshold for recommending surgery in adult patients must therefore involve a careful assessment of symptom burden, functional limitation, and quality of life, weighed against the significantly higher surgical risk that adult patients carry compared to healthy adolescents.

Validated quality of life outcome tools, including disease-specific instruments like the Scoliosis Research Society questionnaires and general instruments like the SF-36, provide objective measures of the impact of scoliosis on a patient's life and can inform and document the quality-of-life rationale for surgical intervention.

COSMETIC CONCERNS — A LEGITIMATE FACTOR

It is appropriate to address directly the role of cosmetic concerns in surgical decision-making, because this is an area that sometimes causes patients to feel uncertain about whether their concerns are being taken seriously.

Visible spinal deformity, including a significant rib hump, uneven shoulders, prominent shoulder blades, and asymmetric waist contour, can have real and significant effects on body image, self-esteem, and quality of life, particularly for adolescents navigating questions of identity and social belonging. Studies measuring quality of life in patients with untreated moderate to severe scoliosis consistently show significantly impaired scores in body image and self-concept domains.

These concerns are legitimate clinical factors. While cosmetic concern alone is generally not considered a sufficient indication for major elective surgery in isolation, it is a meaningful contribution to the overall quality-of-life burden of significant scoliosis, and it is entirely appropriate for patients and families to raise it explicitly in the surgical consultation.

NON-SURGICAL TREATMENTS AND WHY THEY ARE SOMETIMES NOT ENOUGH

A comprehensive understanding of surgical indications requires understanding what non-surgical options exist and why, in certain patients, they are insufficient.

Observation involves regular clinical monitoring with periodic X-rays without active intervention. It is appropriate for mild curves in patients who have finished growing and for mild to moderate curves in growing patients at lower risk of progression. Observation is a clinical choice, not a passive default, and involves active engagement from both the clinical team and the patient.

Bracing is the most evidence-based non-surgical intervention for preventing curve progression in growing patients. The BrAIST trial, a well-conducted randomised controlled trial published in a major medical journal, demonstrated that bracing worn for a mean of 13 hours per day reduced the risk of curve progression to surgical thresholds from 50 percent to 28 percent. Bracing that achieves the recommended 16 to 23 hours per day of wear achieves even better results. Critically, however, bracing does not correct an existing curve. It slows or prevents its growth. And in patients with larger curves, faster-growing patients, or those with poor brace fit or compliance, progression continues despite bracing.

Physiotherapy, and specifically the Schroth method, is a specialised three-dimensional exercise programme developed specifically for scoliosis. Evidence supports its role in improving muscle symmetry, respiratory function, and posture, and it is a valuable complement to bracing. However, physiotherapy cannot structurally correct a curve and is not a surgical alternative once curves have reached a threshold where surgery is clearly indicated.

FROM THE SURGEON'S DESK

The hardest conversations I have are not with patients who arrive angry or frightened, though I have had many of those. The hardest conversations are with patients who ask, quietly and with great seriousness: do I really need this?

My answer is always the same: I would not be recommending surgery if I did not believe the evidence supports it for your specific situation. And then I walk through the evidence with them, not in a lecture, but in a direct, plain-language conversation about what the published data shows for curves like theirs, what the natural history is likely to look like over the coming decades without intervention, and what surgery can realistically achieve.

Most patients, once they understand the trajectory of their untreated curve compared to the evidence-based outcomes of modern surgery, feel more settled about the decision. Knowledge really does reduce fear. And the patient who understands why they are having surgery has a fundamentally different experience of the procedure and its recovery than the patient who is simply told it is necessary and does not fully understand why.

PART TWO

BEFORE SURGERY

CHAPTER FIVE:

CHOOSING THE RIGHT SURGEON AND HOSPITAL

Once surgery has been recommended, one of the most consequential decisions you will make is where to have the procedure performed and who should perform it. This is not a trivial decision to be made primarily on the basis of convenience or familiarity. Scoliosis surgery is one of the technically most demanding procedures in the entire field of orthopaedic and spinal surgery. Outcomes, including the degree of correction achieved, the rate of complications, and the long-term durability of the result, are significantly influenced by the experience and expertise of the surgical team and the institution where the surgery takes place.

This chapter gives you a thorough and practical framework for making this decision well.

WHY SURGEON EXPERIENCE MATTERS SO MUCH IN SCOLIOSIS

In virtually every field of surgery, evidence consistently shows that surgeons and institutions who perform higher volumes of a given procedure achieve better outcomes. This volume-outcome relationship is particularly strong for complex, technically demanding procedures, and scoliosis correction surgery falls squarely into that category.

The reasons are not difficult to understand. A surgeon who performs many scoliosis fusions per year has encountered the full spectrum of anatomical variation, curve complexity, and intraoperative challenges that a lower-volume surgeon may only rarely face. They have developed the fine judgement about screw placement, rod contouring, and correction manoeuvres that can only be built through repetition. They have refined their complication management protocols through experience. Their theatre team works together as a cohesive unit with smooth, efficient communication. Their post-operative care pathway has been refined over hundreds of cases.

Conversely, a surgeon who performs scoliosis fusions infrequently, perhaps a few times per year as part of a general orthopaedic or even general spinal practice, is working in a less familiar territory with each case. Rare complications may be less well-recognised. Intraoperative judgements may be less refined. The cumulative experience that translates into consistently excellent outcomes is, by definition, limited.

This is not a criticism of surgeons who work in general rather than subspecialty practice. It is simply a recognition that scoliosis surgery is a subspecialty procedure that produces the best results in the hands of subspecialists.

WHAT TO LOOK FOR IN A SPINAL SURGEON

Subspecialty training in spinal deformity is the most important credential to look for. Spinal surgery is a broad field that encompasses disc disease, trauma, tumour, infection, and deformity among many other areas. Not all spinal surgeons are equally experienced or trained in deformity correction. The surgeons with the best outcomes in scoliosis are typically those who have completed a dedicated fellowship in spinal deformity, usually one to two years of additional training after completing their primary surgical specialist training, during which they focused specifically on complex spinal reconstruction and deformity correction.

Annual case volume matters. Ask directly how many scoliosis fusions, and specifically how many cases similar to yours, the surgeon performs per year. A surgeon who performs 50 or more spinal deformity cases annually is operating in a very different experience context from one who performs five or ten.

Professional society membership and engagement provide indirect evidence of a surgeon's commitment to staying current with the evidence base in their field. The Scoliosis Research Society is the major international organisation for spinal deformity specialists. Its membership standards include case volume requirements and continuing education. Active participation in professional societies, including presentation of research, involvement in guideline development, and peer review activity, indicates engagement with the highest levels of the specialty.

Communication quality is not a soft or secondary consideration. Your surgeon needs to be able to explain your diagnosis clearly, walk you through the surgical plan in detail, give you honest information about risks and realistic expectations, and be accessible to answer questions before and after surgery. A surgeon who seems rushed, who uses language without explaining it, who dismisses questions as unnecessary, or who presents the plan without inviting your input is not giving you the care you deserve, regardless of their technical ability.

WHAT TO LOOK FOR IN A HOSPITAL OR SURGICAL CENTRE

Dedicated paediatric expertise is essential if the patient is a child or adolescent. Specialist children's hospitals or hospitals with dedicated paediatric spinal deformity programmes have nursing staff, anaesthesiologists, physiotherapists, and intensive care teams who are specifically experienced in caring for young patients undergoing major spinal surgery. Paediatric anaesthesia, pain management, and post-operative nursing care require specific expertise that differs substantially from adult practice.

Routine intraoperative neurophysiological monitoring is non-negotiable for spinal deformity surgery. This involves continuous real-time monitoring of spinal cord and nerve root function throughout the operation. It requires a team of dedicated neurophysiologists, appropriate monitoring equipment, and surgeons who are experienced in responding to monitoring changes intraoperatively. If a surgical centre does not routinely use IONM for scoliosis cases, that is a significant concern.

A comprehensive blood management programme is important for managing the blood loss that accompanies major scoliosis surgery. Hospitals with experience in intraoperative cell salvage, autologous blood donation, and anaesthetic blood conservation strategies are significantly better equipped to manage this aspect of care safely.

A dedicated post-operative care pathway, with specialist nursing staff trained in spinal surgery care, robust pain management protocols, and a physiotherapy team experienced in early post-operative mobilisation after spinal fusion, significantly affects both the safety and the pace of recovery.

Multidisciplinary team working reflects a hospital's commitment to comprehensive care. Complex spinal deformity cases benefit from input not just from the spinal surgeon but from anaesthesiologists with spinal expertise, neurophysiologists, physiotherapists, specialised nurses, and in some cases haematologists, cardiologists, or pulmonologists. Hospitals where these specialists work together in a coordinated way around complex patients produce better outcomes than settings where each specialty acts in isolation.

QUESTIONS TO ASK YOUR SURGEON BEFORE COMMITTING

You have every right, and indeed every reason, to ask your surgeon direct questions before agreeing to a major operation. A good surgeon will answer these questions fully and without defensiveness. Here are the most important ones:

How many scoliosis operations similar to mine do you perform each year? What surgical approach are you planning for my specific curve, and why is that approach appropriate for my case? What degree of correction do you anticipate achieving? What are the most common complications you see in cases like mine, and how do you manage them? Is intraoperative neurophysiological monitoring used throughout the procedure? Who performs the monitoring, and what is the protocol when a signal change is detected? What does the post-operative care pathway look like at this institution? When can I expect to go home, and what support will I need? What is your personal revision rate, and what are the most common reasons your patients require revision?

If a surgeon appears irritated by these questions, provides vague or dismissive answers, or seems to regard your desire for information as an inconvenience, that is important information about the quality of care you are likely to receive.

GETTING A SECOND OPINION

It cannot be emphasised strongly enough that seeking a second opinion before major spinal surgery is not disloyal, not an expression of distrust, and not an unusual or unreasonable thing to do. It is intelligent, responsible patient behaviour, and most experienced spinal surgeons not only accept but actively encourage it.

A second opinion from an appropriately qualified specialist may confirm the recommended approach, which is valuable reassurance. It may offer an alternative surgical plan that differs in technique, approach, or extent, which gives you important comparative information. Or in rare cases, it may suggest that surgery is not yet necessary or appropriate, which is obviously valuable to know. All three outcomes are beneficial.

When arranging a second opinion, bring all imaging studies with you, including the actual films or digital images, not just the written reports. Bring a summary of your clinical history, current medications, and the first surgeon's recommendation. The second surgeon will want to review everything from scratch, which is entirely appropriate.

FROM THE SURGEON'S DESK

When patients ask me what to look for in a surgeon, I give them one piece of advice above all others: find someone who makes you feel informed, not managed.

There is a style of medicine that treats patients as passive recipients of decisions made on their behalf. That approach is wrong, and it is especially wrong in a situation like scoliosis surgery, where the patient and family have to live with the outcome for the rest of their lives.

The surgeon you want is one who takes time with you. Who listens to your concerns before presenting solutions. Who shows you your imaging and explains what it means. Who has a frank conversation about risks without either minimising them or using them as a blunt instrument to pressure a decision. Who acknowledges when evidence is uncertain. Who clearly respects your right to ask questions, to take time to decide, and to seek additional opinions.

Those qualities do not replace technical skill. You need both. But in my experience, the surgeons who take the time to truly inform their patients are also, more often than not, the ones who have the experience and judgement to manage the technical challenges well. The two things tend to go together.

CHAPTER SIX:

PREPARING FOR SURGERY WHAT TO DO BEFORE YOU GO IN

Surgery is not something that simply happens to you. It is something you actively participate in. The decisions you make, the preparations you undertake, and the physical and mental state in which you arrive on the day of the operation all have measurable impacts on your outcomes. The concept of prehabilitation, the work you do before surgery to optimise your readiness for it, is increasingly recognised in the surgical literature as a meaningful contributor to recovery, and this chapter covers every practical aspect of it.

PRE-OPERATIVE MEDICAL ASSESSMENT

Before any major elective operation, your surgical team will arrange a comprehensive pre-operative medical assessment. The purpose of this assessment is threefold: to identify any medical conditions or physiological factors that increase surgical risk, to optimise your health before surgery to the extent possible, and to plan your anaesthetic and post-operative care in the most appropriate way for your individual situation.

Blood tests are a standard component of the pre-operative work-up and typically include a full blood count to assess haemoglobin and platelet levels, a metabolic panel to assess kidney and liver function, a clotting screen to identify any bleeding disorders, and a blood type and cross-match so that compatible blood is available for transfusion if needed during surgery. In specific situations, additional blood tests may be requested, including inflammatory markers in patients with inflammatory conditions, hormonal and nutritional assessments in patients with relevant history, and specific tests related to any known medical conditions.

An electrocardiogram, commonly called an ECG, records the electrical activity of the heart and is routinely performed in adult patients and in younger patients with any cardiac history or symptoms. It identifies rhythm abnormalities, conduction problems, and signs of cardiac strain that might affect anaesthetic management.

Chest X-ray may be requested in adult patients, those with known lung conditions, and patients with large thoracic curves where pulmonary function is a concern. Pulmonary function tests, which measure the volumes and flow rates of air the lungs can move, are specifically indicated in patients with significant thoracic scoliosis where the rib cage deformity may be impairing lung mechanics.

The anaesthetic consultation is one of the most important preoperative appointments. The anaesthetist is the specialist who will be responsible for maintaining your safety and comfort throughout the operation, and their assessment of your fitness for surgery and their planning of the anaesthetic approach is a critical component of the overall care plan. During this consultation, the anaesthetist will review your medical history in detail, discuss any previous anaesthetics and any reactions or difficulties, assess your airway, explain the planned anaesthetic approach, and address any questions or concerns you have about being anaesthetised.

STOPPING AND ADJUSTING MEDICATIONS

Many patients are taking regular medications for chronic conditions, and some of these require adjustment in the period before surgery. This is an area where you must be absolutely proactive and transparent with your surgical and anaesthetic team. Never assume that a medication is safe to continue without checking, and never stop a prescribed medication without medical guidance.

Non-steroidal anti-inflammatory drugs, including ibuprofen, diclofenac, naproxen, and aspirin at anti-inflammatory doses, affect platelet function and increase bleeding risk. They are generally stopped one to two weeks before surgery. Paracetamol is safe to continue.

Anticoagulant medications, including warfarin, rivaroxaban, apixaban, dabigatran, and others used to prevent blood clots, must be carefully managed before surgery. Depending on the specific medication and the reason it is prescribed, the approach may involve stopping the medication several days before surgery with or without bridging anticoagulation. This must be planned in detail with both the prescribing physician and the surgical team.

Herbal and nutritional supplements are frequently overlooked, but several have clinically significant effects on bleeding. Fish oil, vitamin E at high doses, garlic supplements, ginkgo biloba, and St John's Wort all affect platelet function or drug metabolism and should be stopped at least two weeks before surgery.

Diabetes medications require careful management around the time of surgery, as the metabolic stress of the operation affects blood sugar levels and the fasting requirement before surgery disrupts normal meal-time dosing. Insulin-dependent diabetic patients will have a specific perioperative insulin protocol arranged. Patients taking metformin are typically advised to stop it 24 to 48 hours before surgery to reduce the risk of a rare but serious complication associated with combined metformin use and contrast agents.

PHYSICAL PREPARATION — PREHABILITATION

The concept of prehabilitation, preparing the body through exercise and physical optimisation before surgery, is supported by a growing evidence base demonstrating that patients who are fitter at the time of surgery recover more quickly and with fewer complications. Even a few weeks of focused preparation can make a measurable difference.

Cardiovascular fitness directly affects how well the body tolerates the physiological stress of major surgery and anaesthesia. Improved cardiovascular fitness means the heart and lungs can meet the demands of the post-operative period more effectively. Even modest improvements in cardiovascular fitness, achieved through regular walking, swimming, or cycling in the weeks before surgery, are worthwhile.

The muscles around the spine provide important support during the post-operative period. While heavy spinal loading exercises are obviously not appropriate before spinal surgery, gentle core activation and general body conditioning are beneficial. Your physiotherapy team, ideally seen as part of the pre-operative process, can guide you on appropriate exercises.

Respiratory preparation is particularly important for patients with large thoracic curves where lung function may be compromised. Breathing exercises and incentive spirometry, using a device to encourage deep breathing, can improve the baseline lung function and prepare the respiratory muscles for the demands of the post-operative period.

SMOKING — THE MOST IMPORTANT MODIFIABLE RISK FACTOR

If you smoke and you are facing spinal fusion surgery, stopping smoking is the single most impactful thing you can do to improve your surgical outcomes. The evidence on this is stark and unambiguous.

Nicotine and other smoking-related chemicals impair the biological processes of bone healing and fusion in multiple ways. They reduce blood supply to the bone through vasoconstriction of small blood vessels, impair the function of the bone-forming cells called osteoblasts, and promote the activity of the bone-dissolving cells called osteoclasts. The net result is a dramatically higher rate of non-union, the failure of bone graft to fuse, in smokers compared to non-smokers. Studies report non-union rates two to four times higher in smokers than in non-smokers following spinal fusion.

Beyond the specific issue of fusion biology, smoking impairs wound healing by reducing tissue oxygenation, increases the risk of post-operative chest infections, and is associated with higher overall complication rates after major surgery.

Many experienced spinal surgeons will decline to perform elective spinal fusion surgery on active smokers for precisely these reasons. The evidence base for this position is strong. If your surgeon raises this issue with you, please take it seriously. Stopping smoking before surgery, even for just a few weeks, produces measurable biological benefits, and cessation maintained through the recovery period substantially improves the chances of a successful outcome.

NUTRITIONAL OPTIMISATION

Good nutrition in the weeks before surgery provides the biological raw materials needed for tissue repair, immune function, and bone formation. Nutritional deficiencies are more common than many patients realise, particularly among elderly patients, patients with chronic illness, and patients who have poor dietary habits.

Protein is the most important macronutrient for surgical recovery. Every process involved in healing, from collagen synthesis in the wound to bone formation in the fusion mass to immune cell production, depends on adequate protein. The recommended protein intake for patients undergoing major surgery is substantially higher than average dietary consumption. Aim for 1.2 to 1.5 grams of protein per kilogram of body weight per day in the weeks before surgery. For a 70-kilogram patient, this means 84 to 105 grams of protein per day.

Calcium and vitamin D are critical for bone health and the bone fusion process that is the essential biological component of the surgical correction. Many patients are deficient in vitamin D, particularly those who live in regions with limited sunlight, those who spend most of their time indoors, and elderly patients. A simple blood test can assess your vitamin D level. If it is low, supplementation with vitamin D and calcium should begin well before surgery.

Iron is needed for adequate haemoglobin production. Patients who are anaemic before surgery are at higher risk of requiring blood transfusion and of having a more complicated post-operative course. Your pre-operative blood tests will identify any anaemia, and iron supplementation or other treatments will be recommended if needed.

PREPARING YOUR HOME FOR RECOVERY

Thinking carefully about your home environment and making appropriate modifications before surgery significantly reduces stress and difficulty during the recovery period.

The sleeping arrangement is worth careful thought. In the early weeks after surgery, getting in and out of bed requires specific techniques and can be difficult if the bed is very low or very high. A firm mattress at approximately knee height is most suitable. If your bedroom is on an upper floor and negotiating stairs in the early recovery period seems likely to be difficult, consider whether a temporary ground-floor sleeping arrangement is feasible.

Bathroom adaptations improve safety and independence. A handheld shower head, a shower chair or stool, grab rails beside the shower and toilet, a raised toilet seat to reduce the depth of bending required to sit down, and non-slip mats on the bathroom floor are all practical aids that many patients find helpful in the post-operative period.

Clothing strategy simplifies daily routines. Loose elasticated waistbands, front-fastening tops, slip-on shoes, and long-handled devices to help with putting on socks and shoes are all useful in the weeks when bending and reaching are restricted.

Support arrangements are perhaps the most important preparation of all. You will need help at home, particularly in the first two to four weeks after discharge. Identify the people in your life who can provide practical assistance with meals, shopping, transport to appointments, and household tasks. If you live alone or if your usual support network is limited, discuss this with your surgical team's social worker or nurse coordinator before surgery. Unmet support needs at home are a safety risk in the post-operative period.

The practical checklist: medications filled at the pharmacy before going in, easy meals prepared or arranged in advance, household items stored at accessible heights so bending and reaching are minimised, a comfortable chair from which you can rise without difficulty, and entertainment and reading material prepared for what will be a period of limited mobility.

FROM THE SURGEON'S DESK

I am always struck by the difference between patients who arrive for surgery prepared and those who have not thought about it much until the day arrives. It is visible from the moment they come in.

Prepared patients are not necessarily calm. Surgery is a significant event and calm is not always realistic. But they are oriented. They know what the day will look like. They have arranged things at home. They have thought about what they need during recovery. They have a support system in place. And when minor things go differently from expected, as they always do in major surgery, they absorb the adjustment more easily because they were already prepared for uncertainty.

Unprepared patients tend to arrive with a frozen quality. They have been avoiding thinking about it until now, and the unprocessed anxiety surfaces all at once. The recovery, in my observation, tends to be more difficult.

Preparation is not about eliminating all uncertainty. It is about reducing the unnecessary uncertainty, the kind that comes from not knowing what to expect, so that your energy can be directed where it most needs to go: toward healing.

PART THREE

THE SURGERY ITSELF

Chapter Seven:

Nutrition, Sleep, and Mental Preparation Before Surgery

Surgery is a profound physiological event. The body will experience significant physical stress during and after the operation. Blood is lost. Tissues are disrupted. An inflammatory response is mounted. Healing begins. All of these processes demand biological resources, and the body that goes into surgery well-nourished, adequately rested, and psychologically prepared handles these demands more efficiently and recovers more completely than the body that does not.

This chapter focuses on three areas that are frequently underemphasised in standard pre-operative guidance but that have real, measurable impacts on surgical outcomes: nutrition, sleep, and psychological preparation.

NUTRITION IN THE WEEKS BEFORE SURGERY

The relationship between nutritional status and surgical outcomes is one of the most robustly established in the perioperative medicine literature. Patients who are nutritionally deficient at the time of surgery have higher rates of wound complications, longer hospital stays, higher rates of infection, and poorer functional recovery. Conversely, optimising nutrition before surgery produces measurable benefits even over relatively short preparation periods.

Protein — The Essential Building Block

Protein is the fundamental macronutrient for surgical recovery. Every biological process involved in healing requires protein: synthesising collagen for wound repair, building new bone in the fusion mass, producing antibodies for immune defence, repairing damaged muscle fibres, and manufacturing the clotting factors that control bleeding. The recommended protein intake for patients in the pre-operative and post-operative periods is substantially higher than typical dietary consumption, generally 1.2 to 1.5 grams per kilogram of body weight per day.

For perspective, a sedentary adult generally consumes and requires approximately 0.8 grams of protein per kilogram per day. Major surgical patients need 50 to 90 percent more than this. For a 70-kilogram patient, this means aiming for 85 to 105 grams of protein daily, which requires conscious dietary attention.

High-quality protein sources include lean meats such as chicken, turkey, and lean beef, fish and seafood, eggs and dairy products including milk, yoghurt, and cheese, and plant-based sources including legumes, lentils, chickpeas, tofu, and edamame. Distributing protein intake across multiple meals and snacks throughout the day is more effective than attempting to consume the entire daily requirement in one or two sittings, because the body has a limited capacity to use protein efficiently from any single intake.

If dietary protein intake is insufficient, supplemental protein in the form of shakes, powders, or bars can be a practical option. Whey protein supplements, which are derived from dairy, have a particularly favourable amino acid profile for tissue synthesis. Plant-based protein supplements are equally appropriate for those who prefer them.

IRON AND HAEMOGLOBIN

Adequate haemoglobin levels before surgery directly affect how well you tolerate the blood loss that accompanies major spinal surgery. Patients with pre-operative anaemia, low haemoglobin, are more likely to require blood transfusion during or after surgery, and anaemia in the post-operative period prolongs fatigue and slows functional recovery.

Your pre-operative blood tests will identify any anaemia. If your haemoglobin is below the optimal level, your surgical team will recommend treatment, which may include oral iron supplementation, intravenous iron infusion for more severe or treatment-resistant cases, and occasionally erythropoietin injections to stimulate red blood cell production.

Dietary iron is found in two forms. Haem iron, found in red meat, poultry, and fish, is more readily absorbed by the body than non-haem iron, found in plant sources such as spinach, lentils, beans, and fortified cereals. Vitamin C consumed at the same time as non-haem iron enhances its absorption, which is why combining iron-rich plant foods with vitamin C-containing foods is nutritionally advantageous.

VITAMIN D AND CALCIUM FOR BONE FUSION

The surgical outcome depends not only on the technical skill of the surgeon but also on the biological process of bone fusion that occurs in the weeks and months after the operation. This fusion process requires adequate calcium and vitamin D as essential raw materials.

Vitamin D deficiency is remarkably common in the general population, with estimates suggesting that up to 40 to 50 percent of adults in many countries have insufficient levels. Risk factors include limited sun exposure, living at northern latitudes, dark skin pigmentation, obesity, and older age. Vitamin D deficiency significantly impairs bone metabolism and fusion biology. A simple blood test, a 25-hydroxyvitamin D level, can assess your status, and supplementation with vitamin D, typically at a dose of 1000 to 4000 IU daily depending on the degree of deficiency, is safe and effective.

Calcium requirements for adults are generally 1000 to 1200 milligrams per day. Dairy products are the richest dietary sources, but calcium is also found in fortified plant-based milks, canned fish with soft bones, tofu made with calcium sulphate, and green leafy vegetables such as kale and broccoli.

WHAT TO AVOID

Several dietary substances should be reduced or eliminated in the weeks before surgery. Alcohol impairs immune function, increases bleeding risk, disrupts sleep, and impairs wound healing. It should be avoided entirely in at least the two weeks before surgery. Excessive sugar and processed carbohydrates can impair immune function and promote inflammation. A diet emphasising whole foods, lean proteins, vegetables, fruits, and complex carbohydrates is ideal in the preoperative period.

SLEEP — WHY IT MATTERS MORE THAN MOST PATIENTS REALISE

Sleep is not passive. During sleep, the body performs essential maintenance and repair functions. Growth hormone, which plays a critical role in tissue synthesis and repair, is secreted primarily during deep sleep. Immune function is largely regulated during sleep. Emotional processing and cognitive consolidation occur during dreaming. Chronic sleep deprivation before surgery has been shown in multiple studies to increase post-operative pain sensitivity, increase the requirement for pain medications, slow recovery, and impair immune function.

Many patients experience disrupted sleep in the weeks before major surgery, primarily because of anxiety. The mind, at rest in bed without the distraction of daytime activity, tends to revisit fears and worries about the upcoming procedure. This is normal and universal, but it can create a vicious cycle in which anxiety disrupts sleep, sleep deprivation worsens anxiety, and both together reduce psychological resilience going into the operation.

Practical strategies for improving pre-operative sleep include maintaining a consistent sleep schedule, going to bed and rising at the same time every day regardless of whether you feel you have slept well, as regularity supports the circadian rhythm that governs sleep-wake cycles. Limiting screen use for at least one hour before bed reduces exposure to blue-wavelength light, which suppresses melatonin secretion and delays sleep onset. Keeping the bedroom cool, quiet, and dark optimises the sleeping environment. Avoiding caffeine after midday and limiting fluid intake in the evening reduce awakenings.

If you lie awake worrying, a technique called constructive worry can be helpful. This involves setting aside 15 minutes in the early evening to write down everything you are worried about, and beside each worry, write what you will do about it or when you will address it. This offloads the worry from your mind into a written record, which reduces the brain's tendency to rehearse the worries during sleep.

If sleep disruption is severe and persistent, discuss it with your general practitioner or surgical team. In some cases, a short-term course of a sleep aid may be appropriate in the immediate pre-operative period.

PSYCHOLOGICAL PREPARATION — THE EVIDENCE BASE

The psychological dimension of surgical preparation is not soft or ancillary. It is supported by substantial evidence linking pre-operative psychological state to measurable post-operative outcomes. Pre-operative anxiety, in multiple studies, is associated with increased post-operative pain scores, greater opioid analgesic consumption, longer hospital stays, slower return to function, and lower patient satisfaction with outcomes.

Conversely, interventions that reduce pre-operative anxiety produce measurable improvements in all these metrics. The mechanisms are physiological as well as psychological: anxiety activates the sympathetic nervous system and the hypothalamic-pituitary-adrenal axis, raising cortisol and adrenaline levels, which increases inflammation, impairs immune function, and heightens pain sensitivity. Reducing anxiety reduces these physiological effects.

The most powerful pre-operative anxiolytic, meaning anxiety-reducing tool, available to patients is information. This is the foundation on which this entire book is built. Patients who understand their diagnosis, their surgical plan, what the operation involves, and what recovery will look like enter surgery with a fundamentally different psychological profile from those who are going into a largely unknown experience. Known experiences are less frightening than unknown ones, even when the known experience is difficult.

Mindfulness-based practices have the strongest evidence base among specific psychological preparation interventions. Mindfulness meditation involves deliberately directing attention to present-moment experience, including bodily sensations, emotions, and thoughts, with a quality of non-judgmental curiosity rather than reactive distress. Randomised controlled trials have demonstrated that even relatively brief mindfulness programmes in the pre-operative period reduce anxiety, reduce post-operative pain, and reduce analgesic requirements. Well-designed mindfulness apps and online programmes make this accessible to patients who have no prior experience with the practice.

Cognitive reframing is a technique drawn from cognitive-behavioural therapy. Applied to surgical preparation, it involves examining the thoughts and beliefs driving pre-operative anxiety and testing their accuracy. Many patients approach surgery with a narrative of catastrophe: what if something goes wrong, what if the pain is unmanageable, what if I never recover fully. Cognitive reframing involves replacing these catastrophising narratives with more accurate, evidence-based ones: what is the actual probability of serious complications, what do the outcome data show for patients like me, what specific steps are in place to manage any difficulties that arise.

For patients with significant pre-existing anxiety, depression, or previous traumatic medical experiences, pre-operative psychological support from a clinical psychologist or liaison psychiatry service can be transformative. Many hospital systems now incorporate psychological support into prehabilitation programmes for major surgery. If this is not routinely offered at your institution, ask whether it is available.

FROM THE SURGEON'S DESK

I have become increasingly convinced, over the course of my career, that the patient who arrives at surgery in good nutritional shape, reasonably rested, and psychologically prepared heals differently from the patient who does not. Not just in ways that feel subjective, but in measurable, clinical terms.

I now regard pre-operative optimisation as an integral part of the surgical pathway, not an optional add-on. The operation I perform in the theatre is one component of a larger care process that begins weeks before the patient arrives and continues for months after discharge. The outcomes are better when every component is attended to, and nutrition, sleep, and psychological preparation are components that patients have direct control over.

If your team is not talking to you about these things, ask. The conversations are important.

CHAPTER EIGHT:

SURGICAL APPROACHES UNDERSTANDING YOUR OPTIONS

One of the most common sources of confusion for patients is the variety of surgical approaches available for scoliosis correction. Terms like posterior fusion, anterior release, lateral approach, and pedicle subtraction osteotomy appear in consultation letters and surgical plans without adequate explanation, leaving patients uncertain about what is actually being proposed and why. This chapter provides a thorough explanation of the main surgical approaches, what each involves at a practical level, when each is appropriate, and what the key differences between them mean for you as a patient.

THE FUNDAMENTAL GOAL OF ALL SCOLIOSIS SURGERY

Before exploring the different approaches, it is important to establish what all scoliosis surgery, regardless of technique, is trying to achieve. The goals are consistent: to stop curve progression permanently, to correct the deformity in all three planes of the spine, meaning the side-to-side curve, the rotational component, and the sagittal profile, to restore and maintain spinal balance in both the coronal and sagittal planes, to decompress any neural structures that are being compressed by the deformity, and to achieve this correction in a way that will remain durable over the decades of the patient's remaining life.

The different surgical approaches represent different pathways to achieving these goals, each with their own advantages, disadvantages, and specific indications. The choice of approach for any individual patient depends on the type and location of the curve, its flexibility or rigidity, the patient's age and skeletal maturity, associated pathology such as stenosis or disc degeneration, and the surgeon's training and experience.

THE POSTERIOR APPROACH — THE MOST WIDELY USED TECHNIQUE

The posterior approach to the spine is, by a considerable margin, the most commonly employed technique for scoliosis correction in contemporary practice. It is used for the vast majority of adolescent idiopathic scoliosis cases and for many adult deformity cases as well.

As the name indicates, the approach is made from the back of the patient. The patient is positioned lying face-down, in what is called the prone position, on a specially designed operating frame that supports the chest and pelvis while allowing the abdomen to hang free. This free-hanging abdomen position reduces abdominal venous pressure and consequently reduces epidural venous bleeding during the surgical exposure.

A midline incision is made along the length of the spine to be operated on, extending from the upper end vertebra to the lower end vertebra of the planned fusion. The skin and subcutaneous tissues are divided, and the paraspinal muscles are carefully elevated from the posterior bony elements of the spine using a combination of electrocautery and blunt dissection. This exposure reveals the laminae, spinous processes, and transverse processes of the vertebrae to be included in the fusion.

Pedicle screw placement is the next major step and is the foundation of modern posterior scoliosis correction. A pedicle screw is a specially designed titanium screw that is inserted through the pedicle, the bony column connecting the posterior elements to the vertebral body, and driven into the body of the vertebra itself. Because the pedicle traverses the outer cortical shell of the vertebral body, a screw placed accurately through it and anchored in the dense bone of the vertebral body achieves fixation that is extraordinarily strong, resisting forces in all directions.

The technique of pedicle screw placement has been refined considerably over the decades and is now assisted by image-guided navigation systems in many specialist centres. The surgeon uses anatomical landmarks, real-time fluoroscopic imaging, or three-dimensional navigation to guide the precise trajectory of each screw through the narrow pedicle channel. Typical pedicle diameters in the thoracic spine range from 4 to 8 millimetres depending on the level and patient size, which conveys why precision in screw placement is so important.

Once screws have been placed bilaterally at multiple levels throughout the extent of the planned fusion, titanium connecting rods are contoured by hand to match the desired corrected spinal alignment. These rods are inserted into the screw heads and secured. The surgeon then performs a series of carefully controlled manoeuvres to progressively correct the deformity. These typically include rod rotation, in which the rod is rotated within the screw heads to translate the lateral curve into the sagittal plane, derotation manoeuvres to address the axial rotation of the vertebrae, and selective compression and distraction, meaning pushing and pulling between specific screw pairs, to fine-tune the correction and optimise spinal balance.

Throughout all of these correction manoeuvres, the neurophysiology team continuously monitors spinal cord and nerve root function, providing real-time safety feedback to the surgical team.

Once satisfactory correction has been achieved and confirmed on intraoperative imaging, the fusion bed is prepared. This involves decortication, the removal of the outer cortical bone layer from the posterior elements using high-speed burrs and osteotomes, exposing the underlying cancellous bone with its rich blood supply and population of bone-forming cells. Bone graft material is then carefully packed across the decorticated surfaces.

The wound is then closed in layers: the paraspinal muscles are reapproximated over the instrumentation, the deeper fascial layer is closed, the subcutaneous layer is closed, and the skin is closed with sutures, staples, or subcuticular technique. Wound drains may be placed to prevent blood accumulating in the dead space left by the dissection.

Modern posterior scoliosis correction achieves excellent three-dimensional correction and has become the dominant technique because it allows the surgeon to access all segments of the thoracic and lumbar spine through a single approach, with good visualisation and control at every level.

THE ANTERIOR APPROACH

The anterior approach to the spine accesses the vertebrae from the front of the body rather than the back. In the thoracic spine, this typically involves a thoracotomy, an incision through the chest wall with deflation of one lung to access the lateral aspect of the thoracic vertebrae and the discs between them. In the lumbar spine, a retroperitoneal approach through the flank is used, carefully displacing the contents of the abdominal cavity to reach the front of the lumbar vertebrae.

The anterior approach provides direct access to the intervertebral discs and the anterior surface of the vertebral bodies. This is advantageous in situations where the discs themselves need to be removed, such as when a severely degenerated or rigid disc is preventing adequate curve correction, or when the anterior column needs to be structurally supported with cage implants.

Historically, combined anterior and posterior surgery was more commonly used in scoliosis, with an anterior disc release performed on one day followed by posterior instrumentation and fusion on a subsequent day. This two-stage approach could achieve correction of rigid curves that could not be adequately corrected with posterior surgery alone. However, with the significant improvements in posterior correction techniques, particularly the widespread adoption of pedicle screws and the development of powerful correction manoeuvres, the need for routine anterior procedures has decreased substantially. Standalone anterior surgery for scoliosis correction is now much less commonly performed than it was two decades ago.

The anterior approach remains important in specific situations, including selective thoracic fusion for certain curve patterns where anterior disc release genuinely adds correction, correction of some congenital vertebral anomalies where the anterior column pathology is primary, and in combination with posterior surgery for severe rigid adult deformity requiring maximal correction.

The recovery from a thoracotomy is more demanding than from a posterior-only procedure, involving chest wall pain, restriction of breathing movements, and a longer hospital stay. This consideration influences the decision to use an anterior approach.

LATERAL APPROACHES TO THE LUMBAR SPINE

Lateral interbody fusion techniques represent one of the most significant advances in adult spinal surgery over the past two decades. These approaches access the lumbar spine from the patient's side, through the flank, rather than from the back or the front.

The Extreme Lateral Interbody Fusion, known as XLIF, and the Lateral Lumbar Interbody Fusion, or LLIF, approaches use a corridor through the retroperitoneal space and through the psoas muscle to reach the lateral aspect of the lumbar intervertebral disc. Under intraoperative neuromonitoring guidance to protect the nerves that pass through the psoas, the surgeon uses sequential dilators to create a working channel through which the disc can be removed and a structural cage implant placed between the vertebral bodies.

These lateral cage implants can restore disc height, which in turn opens the collapsed intervertebral foramina and decompresses the nerve roots passing through them. The large cage footprint that is possible with a lateral approach supports the vertebral endplates effectively and promotes fusion. The cage can be lordotically shaped, meaning tapered to restore the inward curve of the lumbar spine, which is particularly important for correcting sagittal plane deformity in adult degenerative scoliosis.

Lateral approaches offer several advantages over traditional open posterior surgery. They are significantly less disruptive to the paraspinal muscles because the posterior musculature is not approached at all in the lateral stage. Blood loss is typically less than with open posterior procedures. The large lateral cage provides better disc height restoration and deformity correction at the disc level than is achievable through posterior approaches alone.

However, lateral approaches are almost always combined with posterior screw-rod instrumentation in the same procedure or a staged procedure, because the lateral cage alone does not provide sufficient rotational stability for scoliosis correction. The combination of lateral cages at one or more levels with posterior instrumentation represents a powerful and effective strategy for adult lumbar deformity correction.

The specific risks of the lateral approach include injury to the genitofemoral nerve, which can cause groin and upper thigh numbness or pain, and in rare cases, injury to the nerve roots passing through the psoas muscle. These risks are managed through meticulous use of intraoperative neurological monitoring during the approach.

INSTRUMENTATION IN DETAIL — WHAT GOES INTO THE SPINE

For many patients, one of the more anxiety-provoking aspects of scoliosis surgery is knowing that metal implants will be permanently placed in their spine. Understanding precisely what these implants are, what they do, and what they mean for daily life significantly reduces this understandable concern.

Modern spinal implants for scoliosis are manufactured from titanium alloy, specifically titanium-aluminium-vanadium alloy in most cases. This material was chosen for spinal implants because it combines extraordinary mechanical strength with complete biological compatibility, meaning the body's immune system does not react to it as a foreign material, and it integrates with the surrounding bone without adverse reaction. Titanium is also essentially non-ferromagnetic, meaning it does not significantly interact with the magnetic fields used in MRI scanning, and it does not set off standard airport metal detector systems in the way that older steel implants sometimes did.

Pedicle screws are the primary anchoring elements and have been described in the context of the posterior approach above. Their design has evolved considerably over the decades. Modern pedicle screws feature polyaxial heads, meaning the screw head can pivot in multiple directions, which allows it to accept the connecting rod even when the rod's trajectory does not perfectly align with the screw's axis. This flexibility greatly facilitates rod insertion in the context of a deformed spine.

Connecting rods link the pedicle screws along the length of the fusion and transmit the corrective forces between them. Modern rods are available in different diameters and alloys to provide different combinations of stiffness and strength depending on the surgical requirements. In some situations, two rods are used on each side of the spine, so-called dual-rod constructs, to increase the rigidity and load-sharing capacity of the construct.

Cross-connectors are short bridges placed perpendicular to the connecting rods, linking the rods on the two sides of the spine to each other. They add torsional rigidity to the construct and are particularly important in long-segment fusions.

Hooks and sub-laminar wires were the primary fixation devices used in scoliosis surgery before pedicle screws became widely adopted. They remain in use in specific situations, particularly at the uppermost levels of thoracic fusions where pedicle screw placement may be more technically challenging, and they can be combined with pedicle screws in hybrid constructs.

BONE GRAFT — THE BIOLOGY OF FUSION

The metal instrumentation corrects and holds the spinal alignment, but the biological process of bone fusion across the instrumented segments is what makes the correction permanent. This distinction is critical: the instrumentation is temporary in the biological sense, meaning it bears load while fusion is occurring, but it is not designed to bear cyclical loading indefinitely without biological support. A spine that is instrumented but not fused will eventually experience implant fatigue and failure. A spine that is instrumented and solidly fused is a permanent, stable construct.

Bone graft refers to the biological material used to stimulate and provide the scaffold for new bone formation across the fusion. Several options exist and are frequently used in combination.

Autologous bone graft, bone taken from the patient's own body, is the biological gold standard for spinal fusion because it contains all three components needed for optimal bone formation: osteogenic cells which are the bone-forming cells themselves, osteoinductive factors which are the chemical signals that stimulate surrounding cells to become bone-forming cells, and osteoconductive scaffold which is the physical framework on which new bone grows.

In modern posterior scoliosis surgery, large amounts of local autograft are routinely available from the posterior elements that are removed and prepared during the surgical exposure. Bone chips removed from the spinous processes, laminae, and facet joints during the decortication of the fusion bed provide substantial local autograft that is immediately placed across the prepared fusion surfaces.

Allograft bone, derived from processed cadaveric donors through bone banks, is commonly used to supplement local autograft, providing additional volume of osteoconductive scaffold without the need for a separate donor site harvest. Allograft bone undergoes rigorous processing to eliminate infectious agents and ensure safety.

Bone morphogenetic proteins, commonly abbreviated to BMPs, are naturally occurring proteins in the body that are among the most potent stimulators of bone formation known. Recombinant human BMP-2 is available as a surgical adjunct and is used in selected cases where the risk of non-union is elevated, such as in smokers, diabetic patients, patients requiring revision surgery, or patients with very long fusions where achieving solid bone formation across all levels is biologically challenging.

The process of solid bone fusion is not rapid. Radiographic evidence of bridging bone across the fusion segments typically becomes visible on X-ray at 6 to 12 months. Solid mature fusion, confirmed by CT scanning, is generally achieved at 12 to 18 months, though this varies considerably between patients depending on age, health, nutritional status, and the biological variables that govern bone healing.

FROM THE SURGEON'S DESK

When I describe the instrumentation to patients, I often see a moment of unease at the description of metal implants being permanently placed in the spine. It is a completely understandable reaction.

What I tell patients is this. Those implants are not a foreign intrusion in the way that a splinter is a foreign body, something the body is trying to reject and expel. They are a scaffold, a precise engineering framework that holds the spine in the corrected alignment while the body's own biology does the real and permanent work of healing. Once fusion is complete, the bone that has grown across the fusion segments and around the implants has integrated them into the structure of the spine. The rods and screws become part of the architecture.

The titanium we use is extraordinary material. Lightweight, biocompatible, corrosion-resistant, and stronger in relevant loading conditions than the bone it supplements. Patients with well-fused scoliosis corrections go on to live fully normal, active lives. The hardware does not hold them back.

CHAPTER NINE:

THE LATEST ADVANCES — WHAT MODERN SURGERY LOOKS LIKE

Scoliosis surgery has undergone a profound transformation over the past two to three decades. Techniques that were experimental a generation ago are now established practice. Technologies that did not exist when many adult scoliosis patients were first diagnosed have fundamentally changed what is achievable in terms of correction, safety, and recovery. Understanding these advances is not merely interesting background knowledge. It is directly relevant to the options available to you as a patient and to the conversations you will have with your surgical team.

MINIMALLY INVASIVE POSTERIOR SURGERY

Traditional posterior scoliosis surgery requires a significant exposure of the spine through a midline incision extending the full length of the planned fusion. While this approach provides excellent visualisation and allows all the correction manoeuvres needed, it involves considerable disruption of the paraspinal musculature.

Minimally invasive surgical techniques for the posterior spine use tubular retractors and percutaneous screw insertion systems to place implants and perform limited corrections through much smaller incisions, with significantly reduced disruption of the paraspinal muscles. Rather than reflecting the muscles away from the spine over the full length of the fusion, these techniques use sequential dilators to create a muscle-splitting corridor through which instruments are passed.

The clinical benefits are meaningful. Less muscle disruption translates to less post-operative pain from the wound itself, reduced blood loss, shorter hospital stay, and in many cases faster return to normal activities. Patients who undergo minimally invasive posterior procedures often report that their surgical wound discomfort is less than they expected.

However, there are important limitations. Minimally invasive approaches are most applicable to less severe deformities where the correction required is modest, and where the number of levels to be fused is relatively limited. Complex deformities requiring large corrections, significant rotational correction, or extensive fusion constructs are generally not amenable to fully minimally invasive techniques because the necessary correction manoeuvres require the direct access and force application that only open exposure provides. The choice between open and minimally invasive approaches should always be based on what gives the best outcome for the specific patient, not on the perception that minimally invasive is inherently preferable.

VERTEBRAL BODY TETHERING — THE NON-FUSION ALTERNATIVE

Vertebral Body Tethering, abbreviated to VBT and sometimes called anterior vertebral body tethering or spine tethering, represents one of the most conceptually innovative advances in scoliosis surgery in recent decades. It offers a non-fusion surgical option that is particularly applicable to a specific subset of adolescent patients with idiopathic scoliosis.

The biological principle underlying VBT is the Hueter-Volkmann law, a fundamental principle of bone physiology established in the 19th century and extensively validated since. This law states that compression across a growth plate slows growth on the compressed side, while tension, or distraction force, accelerates growth on the stretched side. Bone responds dynamically to the mechanical forces acting across growth plates, and this response underlies much of normal skeletal development and many growth-related conditions.

In VBT surgery, this principle is exploited to correct scoliosis using growth rather than fighting it. The surgical approach is performed thoracoscopically, meaning through small ports placed between the ribs, with a camera providing visualisation. The deflated lung is gently retracted to access the lateral aspect of the thoracic vertebrae and the discs between them. Screws are placed into the vertebral bodies on the convex, or outer, side of the scoliotic curve. A strong, flexible cord, the tether, typically made of high-strength polyethylene, is then threaded through the screw heads and tensioned.

When the tether is tensioned, it creates a compressive force across the growth plates on the convex side of the curve, and a tensile force on the concave side. Over time, as the patient continues to grow, the compressed convex side grows more slowly than the tension-stimulated concave side. This differential growth progressively corrects the curve, using the patient's own growth as the corrective mechanism. The result, when the technique works as intended, is a corrected and balanced spine that has retained its normal segmental mobility because no fusion has been performed.

The preservation of spinal motion is the most compelling advantage of VBT over fusion. A teenager who undergoes fusion of 10 or more thoracic vertebral levels will have significantly reduced thoracic spinal mobility for the rest of their life. A teenager who undergoes VBT and achieves good correction retains nearly normal spinal flexibility, which has implications for long-term function and quality of life, particularly for patients with aspirations toward high-level sport, dance, or other activities requiring spinal mobility.

However, VBT is not suitable for all patients and carries its own specific set of limitations and risks that patients must understand clearly. The most important limitation is that the technique depends on growth. It is not suitable for patients who have completed or nearly completed skeletal growth, because there is no growth force to exploit. The ideal candidate is a growing adolescent, typically Risser 0 to 2, with significant growth remaining, a curve in the range of approximately 40 to 65 degrees, good curve flexibility, and an anatomically suitable curve pattern.

The revision rate following VBT, for reasons including over-correction, under-correction, or tether breakage, is higher than after traditional fusion in published series. The long-term data beyond 5 to 10 years are still accumulating, which means some uncertainty about very long-term outcomes exists in a way that is not the case for fusion, which has decades of follow-up data. These are honest limitations that patients considering VBT should discuss thoroughly with their surgeon.

COMPUTER-ASSISTED NAVIGATION AND ROBOTIC SYSTEMS

Among the most transformative technological advances in spinal surgery is the development of computer-assisted surgical navigation and, building on this, robotic surgical assistance platforms. These systems have fundamentally changed the precision with which spinal implants can be placed and the safety profile of complex spinal deformity surgery.

In traditional pedicle screw placement, the surgeon relies on anatomical landmarks visible at surgery, supplemented by two-dimensional fluoroscopic imaging, to guide the trajectory of each screw through the pedicle. This requires deep three-dimensional anatomical knowledge, refined spatial reasoning, and considerable experience. Even in skilled hands, screw malposition rates in the literature range from approximately 5 to 20 percent depending on how malposition is defined and the experience of the surgical team.

Computer-assisted navigation systems use pre-operative CT data to build a three-dimensional digital model of the patient's spine. Intraoperatively, this model is registered to the patient's actual anatomy using reference markers attached to the surgical field and tracked by an infrared camera system. The surgeon's instruments are similarly tracked, so their precise position within the three-dimensional anatomical model is known and displayed on a monitor in real time. This allows the surgeon to plan and execute screw trajectories with reference to the complete three-dimensional anatomy rather than the limited view available through direct visualisation and two-dimensional fluoroscopy.

Studies consistently show that navigated screw placement reduces the rate of clinically significant screw malposition compared to conventional techniques, with some large series reporting malposition rates below 2 percent with navigation compared to 5 to 15 percent with conventional technique. This improvement in accuracy is particularly meaningful in scoliosis, where the rotated and curved vertebrae present abnormal anatomy that can be deceptive when relying on conventional surface landmarks.

Robotic surgical systems take computer-assisted navigation a step further by adding a robotic arm to the workflow. After the surgeon has planned all screw trajectories in the navigation system, the robotic arm positions a guide sleeve at the precise entry point and along the precise planned trajectory for each screw. The surgeon then places the screw through this precisely positioned guide. This further reduces the reliance on freehand technique and translates the pre-operative plan into the actual operation with exceptional consistency.

Radiation exposure for the surgical team, which is a meaningful long-term occupational health concern for surgeons who perform fluoroscopy-guided procedures throughout their careers, is significantly reduced with navigation systems, because far less real-time fluoroscopy is needed when instrument positions are known through the navigation tracking.

INTRAOPERATIVE NEUROPHYSIOLOGICAL MONITORING

No advance in scoliosis surgery safety has had a more profound impact than the routine use of intraoperative neurophysiological monitoring throughout the entire procedure. This technology provides a continuous, real-time assessment of spinal cord and nerve root function during surgery, serving as an early warning system that allows the surgical team to detect and respond to any compromise of neurological function before it becomes a permanent deficit.

IONM uses two principal monitoring modalities that assess the integrity of different neural pathways. Somatosensory evoked potentials are generated by applying electrical stimuli to peripheral nerves, typically the posterior tibial nerves at the ankles, and recording the electrical response in the brain using scalp electrodes. The signal must travel up the peripheral nerve, through the dorsal columns of the spinal cord, to the cortex. Any disruption of this pathway, from stretch or compression of the spinal cord, results in a decrease in the amplitude or an increase in the latency of the recorded signal that the neurophysiologist can detect.

Motor evoked potentials test the integrity of the motor pathways. Transcranial magnetic or electrical stimulation of the motor cortex of the brain generates a signal that travels down the corticospinal tracts of the spinal cord and out to the muscles of the legs, where the response is recorded as muscle electromyographic activity. Monitoring

MEPs tests whether motor commands from the brain can reach the muscles through the spinal cord, which is the most direct test of the pathways at greatest risk during correction manoeuvres.

The neurophysiologist, a specialist in neural monitoring, continuously interprets both SSEP and MEP data throughout the operation and reports the status to the surgical team at regular intervals, and immediately if any significant change is detected. Alert criteria, including a 50 percent decrease in SSEP amplitude or any loss of MEP responses, trigger an immediate halt in the surgical manoeuvre that may be causing the change, and a series of corrective steps to restore normal neurological function.

The impact of universal IONM on neurological outcomes from scoliosis surgery has been dramatic. The incidence of permanent neurological deficit, including significant weakness or paralysis, after scoliosis surgery has fallen substantially since IONM became routine practice. Performing scoliosis surgery without continuous, full-modality IONM is now considered below the standard of care at specialist centres.

THREE-DIMENSIONAL PLANNING AND PATIENT-SPECIFIC IMPLANTS

Advances in imaging technology, computational modelling, and additive manufacturing, meaning three-dimensional printing, have begun to transform the planning and execution of complex spinal deformity surgery.

Sophisticated surgical planning software now allows the surgical team to import a patient's pre-operative CT data, build a three-dimensional virtual model of the deformed spine, and simulate the proposed surgical correction. The surgeon can virtually place screws, position rods, and model the expected correction before the patient reaches the operating table. This simulation capability allows the team to identify potential difficulties, optimise the surgical plan, and select the most appropriate implant sizes and configurations in advance.

For the most complex cases, three-dimensional printing technology can produce a physical replica of the patient's spine from the CT data. The surgical team can handle this model, plan the approach, and even perform rehearsal screw placements on the model before surgery. While not yet standard practice for routine cases, this technology is genuinely transformative for the most challenging deformities.

FROM THE SURGEON'S DESK

When patients ask me what has changed most in scoliosis surgery over my career, the answer is not a single technology or technique. It is precision. Everything about modern scoliosis surgery is more precise than it was a generation ago: more precise implant placement, more precise deformity correction, more precise biological understanding of fusion and growth modulation, more precise real-time safety monitoring of the nervous system.

Precision reduces risk. Precision improves correction. Precision builds on itself through training and technology in ways that continue to advance outcomes with each passing decade.

When I place a navigated screw guided by a three-dimensional map of the patient's specific anatomy, I am benefiting from the work of thousands of surgeons, engineers, and researchers who came before me. That accumulated expertise is embedded in the technology, the technique, and the training programme through which I and my colleagues learned. Patients who come to specialist centres are the beneficiaries of that collective effort, and I believe the outcomes they achieve reflect that.

CHAPTER TEN:

PAEDIATRIC VS. ADULT SCOLIOSIS SURGERY — KEY DIFFERENCES

Scoliosis surgery is not a single operation with a standardised approach applied uniformly across all patients. The goals, risks, technical approaches, recovery, and long-term considerations differ substantially depending on the age of the patient, the type of scoliosis, and the specific clinical situation. This chapter outlines the most important differences between scoliosis surgery in children and adolescents compared to adults, helping patients and families understand which considerations are most relevant to their situation.

ADOLESCENT IDIOPATHIC SCOLIOSIS — THE YOUNG PATIENT

Adolescent idiopathic scoliosis surgery is in many ways the most favourable surgical scenario in scoliosis. Patients are young and otherwise healthy, with excellent cardiovascular and respiratory reserves and strong capacity for healing and recovery. The spine is still moderately flexible, allowing good correction. The bones are healthy and dense, providing strong screw purchase. The biological capacity for fusion is robust.

The goals of surgery in adolescent idiopathic scoliosis are to correct the curve to the maximum safely achievable degree, preventing future progression while restoring the best possible balance and alignment. Curve correction rates of 60 to 75 percent of the original Cobb angle are routinely achieved in adolescent idiopathic scoliosis with modern posterior techniques, and these corrections are well-maintained in long-term follow-up studies.

The primary surgeon-level decision in adolescent idiopathic scoliosis surgery is determining the extent of the fusion, specifically how many vertebral levels to include. The fundamental principle is to fuse as few levels as necessary to achieve stable correction while maintaining as much unfused mobile spine as possible. Every unfused mobile level retained preserves useful spinal motion and reduces long-term stress on the unfused segments. However, fusing too few levels risks residual imbalance or curve recurrence. Determining the optimal fusion levels requires detailed pre-operative analysis of the curve pattern, flexibility, and balance parameters, and is one of the key areas where surgical experience and expertise make a significant difference to outcomes.

EARLY ONSET SCOLIOSIS — THE VERY YOUNG CHILD

Scoliosis developing before the age of five years presents challenges that are fundamentally different from those of adolescent scoliosis. At this stage of life, the thoracic cage and the lungs it contains are in a critical phase of development. The alveoli, the microscopic air sacs that are the functional units of lung gas exchange, are still multiplying during the first years of life. The total number of alveoli a person will ever have is largely determined by the age of approximately seven or eight years.

Rigid spinal fusion of the thoracic spine in a very young child would prevent the normal growth and expansion of the thoracic cage, severely limiting alveolar development and potentially causing a devastating condition called thoracic insufficiency syndrome, in which the thorax cannot support normal breathing. This risk has driven the development of an entirely different surgical philosophy for early onset scoliosis: growth-friendly surgery.

Growth-friendly surgical strategies aim to control the scoliotic curve and prevent its progression while allowing the thoracic cage and lungs to continue their normal development. Definitive fusion is deliberately deferred until the child is sufficiently mature, typically in late childhood or early adolescence.

Traditional growing rods are implants anchored at two points, one above and one below the curve, connected by rods that cross the deformity without being attached to the intervening vertebrae. At approximately every six months, the patient undergoes a short surgical procedure under general anaesthesia to lengthen the rods, maintaining control of the curve while allowing height growth. The obvious disadvantage is the requirement for repeated anaesthetics and procedures over what may be a period of five or more years.

Magnetically controlled growing rods represent a significant advance over traditional growing rods. These devices contain a small internal motor that can be activated by an external magnet applied to the patient's back in a clinic setting, without any anaesthetic or surgical procedure. The motor distally translates the rod, elongating it and maintaining the correction. Patients return to clinic every three months, and the rod lengthening takes approximately five minutes with no patient discomfort. This technology has transformed the experience of growing rod management for children and families.

ADULT SCOLIOSIS — A SUBSTANTIALLY DIFFERENT CHALLENGE

Adult scoliosis surgery is substantially more complex than adolescent scoliosis surgery across virtually every dimension. This is not a value judgement about the relative importance of the two groups of patients. It is a clinical reality that has direct implications for surgical planning, expected outcomes, and the risk-benefit calculation that must be made for each patient.

The biological challenges are significant. Adult bone is less metabolically active than adolescent bone, and the biological capacity for fusion is correspondingly reduced. The discs between the vertebrae have degenerated and have reduced height, which changes the mechanical environment for the fusion. Osteoporosis, which becomes increasingly prevalent with advancing age, further compromises bone quality and screw fixation strength.

The structural challenges are equally significant. Adult curves have typically been present for decades and have become substantially more rigid than equivalent curves in adolescents. The soft tissue structures, discs, ligaments, facet joint capsules, have adapted to the deformed position and resist correction. This rigidity may require additional surgical steps to achieve meaningful correction, including osteotomies, which are controlled bony cuts that allow segments of the spine to be repositioned.

There are several types of osteotomy used in adult spinal deformity surgery, each providing different amounts of correction and carrying different levels of surgical risk.

A Smith-Petersen osteotomy, also called a posterior column osteotomy, involves removing bone from the posterior elements of a vertebra to allow controlled closure of the gap and extension of the spine at that level. It can be performed at multiple levels and provides approximately 10 to 15 degrees of correction per level when used in the lumbar spine for sagittal balance correction.

A pedicle subtraction osteotomy is a more powerful but technically demanding procedure in which the entire posterior elements, the pedicles, and a wedge of vertebral body are removed, allowing the spine to close down at that level and providing 30 to 40 degrees of sagittal correction in a single level. It is used for more severe sagittal imbalance but carries higher surgical risk due to the greater blood loss and spinal cord exposure involved.

A vertebral column resection is the most radical osteotomy type, involving complete removal of one or more vertebrae to allow dramatic correction of both coronal and sagittal deformity in severe, rigid curves. It is reserved for the most complex deformities and carries the highest risk of all osteotomy procedures.

OSTEOPOROSIS — THE CRITICAL COMPLICATING FACTOR IN OLDER ADULTS

Among the challenges of adult scoliosis surgery, osteoporosis deserves particular emphasis because it is both common and profoundly affects surgical planning and outcomes.

When a pedicle screw is placed in a vertebra with normal bone density, it achieves excellent purchase, meaning the screw is firmly held in the bone and can transmit significant corrective and stabilising forces. When the same screw is placed in osteoporotic bone, with its reduced mineral content and compromised structural integrity, the purchase achieved is substantially weaker. This has direct consequences for the stability of the construct and the risk of complications including screw loosening, progressive loss of correction, and in the most severe cases, the screw cutting through the weakened bone, a complication called pullout or toggling.

The management of osteoporosis in surgical candidates includes a baseline bone density assessment using a DEXA scan, ideally performed well before surgery so that results are available to inform planning. Medical treatment for osteoporosis should be initiated where appropriate, though some osteoporosis medications require weeks to months before they significantly affect bone density and microstructure.

Intraoperatively, several strategies can augment fixation in osteoporotic bone. Cement augmentation of pedicle screws involves injecting polymethylmethacrylate bone cement through the screw or through a separate channel into the surrounding vertebral body before or after screw placement. The cement hardens around the screw and dramatically increases its pullout strength. Longer fusion constructs that distribute load across more fixation points, and the use of hooks in addition to screws at key levels, also improve construct stability in osteoporotic patients.

FROM THE SURGEON'S DESK

Adult spinal deformity surgery is, in my clinical view, among the most technically and physiologically demanding operations in all of elective surgery. The patients are older and carry more medical risk. The anatomy is complex and often distorted by decades of degenerative change. The operations are longer. The blood loss is greater. The margin for technical error is narrower. The recovery is slower and more arduous.

I say this not to alarm patients or their families, but to explain clearly why the choice of surgeon and institution is even more critical for adult deformity cases than for adolescent cases. An experienced surgeon at a specialist centre with robust multidisciplinary support produces outcomes for complex adult deformity that simply cannot be replicated in a lower-volume or less-specialised setting.

If you are an adult being told you need major spinal deformity surgery, please take seriously the importance of seeking out the most experienced team available for your case. The investment in finding the right place to have this operation is fully justified by the difference in outcomes it makes.

CHAPTER ELEVEN:

THE DAY OF SURGERY — WHAT TO EXPECT

For most patients, the day of surgery is the moment of greatest anxiety in the entire journey. Not knowing what the day will look like, what being anaesthetised feels like, what you will be aware of, and how you will feel when you wake up are all powerful sources of fear. This chapter provides a detailed, honest account of the day from arrival to the recovery room, because knowing what to expect is the single most effective way to reduce the fear of not knowing.

FASTING BEFORE SURGERY

The requirement to fast before surgery is one of the first practical instructions you will receive. Current guidelines in most institutions follow evidence-based fasting protocols that are less restrictive than the traditional midnight-nothing-by-mouth rule. You are generally permitted to drink clear fluids, including water, black tea or black coffee without milk, and clear apple juice, up until two hours before your scheduled surgery time. Solid food and milk-containing drinks should be avoided from six hours before surgery.

These fasting requirements exist because of the risk of aspiration, which is the entry of stomach contents into the airway under anaesthesia. While aspiration is uncommon with modern anaesthetic practice, its consequences can be serious, and fasting reduces the volume of gastric contents to the minimum possible at the time of induction of anaesthesia.

If you have diabetes or any condition that affects how your body responds to fasting, you will receive specific guidance from your anaesthetist about how to manage your condition during the fasting period. Never adjust insulin or other medications without explicit guidance from your medical team.

ARRIVING AT THE HOSPITAL

You will typically be asked to arrive at the hospital one to two hours before your scheduled operation time. This pre-operative window allows for administrative check-in, pre-operative nursing assessment, consent confirmation, preparation, and the inevitable small delays that occur in busy surgical environments.

Pack a small bag with what you will need for your hospital stay. Comfortable loose clothing for when you are mobilising after surgery, your toiletries, any personal items that comfort you, and phone and charger are the practical essentials. Leave jewellery, valuables, and significant amounts of cash at home.

On arrival at the pre-admission or pre-operative ward, a nurse will check your vital signs, confirm your name and date of birth and the procedure you are having, review your medical history and medications, and verify that you have followed the fasting instructions. An intravenous cannula will be placed, usually in the back of the hand or the forearm, through which fluids and medications will be given.

You will be asked to change into a hospital gown. If you are having a posterior procedure, you may also be asked to shower with an antiseptic wash the morning of surgery to reduce the bacterial load on the skin and minimise infection risk.

PRE-OPERATIVE MARKING AND FINAL CONSENT

Before you go to theatre, your surgeon will usually visit you in the pre-operative area to confirm the surgical plan and sign any required marking or documentation. In some institutions, the operative site is marked with a skin marker as part of the safe surgery protocol.

This is your last opportunity before the anaesthetic to ask any questions that have remained on your mind. Do not feel that the process is too far advanced to raise a concern. Every legitimate question deserves an answer before you undergo anaesthesia, and a surgeon who is unwilling to take a few minutes for this is not providing the standard of care you deserve.

THE ANAESTHETIC IN DETAIL

General anaesthesia for scoliosis surgery means you will be completely unconscious throughout the entire procedure, with no awareness, no pain, and no memory of the operation. The prospect of being unconscious can be frightening for some patients, and understanding the process can help.

You will be brought to the anaesthetic room, immediately adjacent to the operating room. Your anaesthetist will be there to receive you. Monitoring electrodes for the ECG and oxygen saturation will be attached, and your blood pressure cuff will be positioned.

Induction of anaesthesia, the process of going to sleep, is accomplished by injecting anaesthetic medications through your intravenous cannula. The onset is extremely rapid, typically within 20 to 30 seconds. Most patients describe the sensation as a feeling of warmth or slight dizziness, followed almost immediately by unconsciousness. There is no frightening transition; the world simply becomes absent.

Once you are unconscious, the anaesthetist places an endotracheal tube through your mouth and into your trachea to maintain a secure airway and allow mechanical ventilation of your lungs throughout the procedure. You are then positioned on the operating frame and surgical preparation of the skin is performed.

Anaesthesia is maintained throughout the procedure using a combination of intravenous agents and inhaled gases. Your anaesthetist monitors every aspect of your physiology continuously throughout the operation: heart rate, blood pressure, oxygen levels, carbon dioxide levels, temperature, depth of anaesthesia, and urine output, among other parameters. Their role, present beside you for the entire duration of the procedure, is your physiological guardian.

Waking from anaesthesia at the end of surgery is gradual. The anaesthetic agents are discontinued, the effects wear off over minutes, and consciousness returns. Most patients experience this as a gentle emergence, though disorientation and grogginess are common and normal. You may have a sore throat from the endotracheal tube. You may feel cold, or nauseous, or confused about where you are. These are all normal and temporary.

POSITIONING AND INTRAOPERATIVE EVENTS

Scoliosis surgery is typically performed with the patient in the prone position, lying face-down on a specially padded operating frame. Careful attention is given to every pressure point on the body to prevent pressure injury during what may be a procedure lasting four to eight hours or more. The eyes are protected to prevent corneal injury. The shoulders and arms are positioned carefully to protect the brachial plexus nerves. The abdomen hangs free of the frame to reduce venous pressure.

Intraoperatively, your safety is attended to by the entire team working in coordination. The cell salvage machine collects blood lost during surgery, processes it, and re-infuses it into your circulation through a separate intravenous line. Your temperature is actively managed to prevent hypothermia, which slows clotting and impairs immune function. Compression stockings or pneumatic calf compression devices reduce the risk of deep vein thrombosis.

The neurophysiology team monitors your SSEP and MEP signals continuously throughout the operation. Every 15 to 20 minutes, and immediately if a surgical manoeuvre might affect neural function, the neurophysiologist reports the status of your monitoring to the surgical team. If a signal change occurs, the team responds immediately with a protocol designed to identify the cause and restore normal monitoring before any permanent injury occurs.

WAKING UP — THE RECOVERY ROOM

When surgery is complete, you will be moved to the post-anaesthetic care unit, commonly called the recovery room. This is a dedicated area immediately adjacent to the operating rooms, staffed by specially trained nurses whose sole responsibility is the monitoring and immediate post-operative care of patients emerging from anaesthesia.

Pain management will already be underway before you fully wake. Analgesic medications will have been given by the anaesthetist at the end of surgery. You may have a patient-controlled analgesia pump connected to your IV line, allowing you to give yourself small supplementary doses of painkiller by pressing a button within the limits of a safety programme.

You may have a urinary catheter in place, a thin tube draining urine from the bladder, which is standard for major spinal surgery and avoids any need to manage urination during the immediate post-operative period when mobility is restricted. You will likely have wound drains, soft plastic tubes placed in the wound to allow any accumulated blood to drain rather than pool under the skin. You will be connected to monitoring equipment tracking your vital signs.

A nurse will be assigned specifically to you during your time in the recovery room, assessing your level of consciousness, pain, vital signs, and neurological function at frequent intervals. Neurological checks, asking you to move your toes and feet and assessing sensation in the legs, are performed as soon as you are conscious enough to cooperate with them. These checks confirm that neurological function is intact in the post-operative period.

FROM THE SURGEON'S DESK

The thing I want patients to understand most about the day of surgery is that they are not alone in that operating room. Surrounding them is a team of professionals whose complete and undivided attention, for the entire duration of the procedure, is focused on that patient.

I have performed hundreds of these operations. Every one of them receives identical preparation and care. The surgical plan has been reviewed. The imaging has been studied. The potential challenges have been anticipated. The equipment has been checked. The neurophysiology team knows the baseline signals for this patient. The anaesthetist knows the medical history and has planned the anaesthetic accordingly.

The patient is unconscious, but they are not alone. They are in the most attentive, coordinated, technically sophisticated care they have perhaps ever received. Knowing that, truly believing it, can be a genuine source of comfort in the anxious days before surgery.

PART FOUR

RECOVERY

Chapter Twelve:

The First Days — Hospital Recovery

The first days after scoliosis surgery are a period of transition, from the completed operation to the beginning of recovery. They are simultaneously a time of significant physical demand and, for many patients, surprising achievement. This chapter covers everything that happens from the recovery room through the first few days on the ward, what to expect, what is normal, what requires concern, and how to be an active participant in your own early recovery.

THE RECOVERY ROOM — THE FIRST HOURS

Your time in the recovery room will typically last one to four hours, depending on how the anaesthetic wears off, how your pain is initially controlled, and your overall physiological stability. During this time, the nursing team is focused on managing any immediate complications, establishing adequate pain control, monitoring your neurological function, and ensuring that your vital signs are stable before you are transferred to the ward.

Pain in the immediate post-operative period varies considerably between patients and is influenced by many factors including the extent of surgery, individual pain sensitivity, pre-operative expectations, and the specific analgesic protocol used. Modern post-operative pain management is multimodal, meaning it uses several different medication classes simultaneously to target pain through multiple physiological mechanisms, achieving better overall control with lower doses of any single agent.

The multimodal analgesic protocol typically includes paracetamol given around the clock as a baseline analgesic. Opioid medications, such as morphine or oxycodone, are used for moderate to severe breakthrough pain and may be delivered via patient-controlled analgesia pump. Nerve-modulating medications such as gabapentin or pregabalin address the neuropathic pain component. Where surgeons use wound infiltration with local anaesthetic at wound closure, this provides additional early pain relief specifically at the wound site.

The goal of pain management is not the complete elimination of pain, which is rarely achievable after major surgery, but rather pain control that allows adequate rest, deep breathing, and participation in early physiotherapy activities. A pain score in the range of three to four out of ten, meaning discomfort that is present but manageable, is a realistic and appropriate initial target.

Neurological checks are performed at regular intervals in the recovery room. The nurse will ask you to move your toes and feet, assess the strength of ankle and knee movements, and check sensation in your legs. These checks are important and should be cooperated with even when you feel drowsy or uncomfortable. Any new neurological abnormality detected in this period triggers an immediate review by the surgical team.

Nausea is a common early post-operative experience, related to both the anaesthetic agents and the opioid pain medications. Anti-nausea medications are routinely prescribed and given preventively. If nausea is distressing, inform the nursing staff, as additional medications or adjustment of the analgesic regimen can often provide relief.

TRANSFER TO THE WARD

Once the immediate post-operative recovery criteria have been met, including stable vital signs, adequate pain control, and no immediate complications, you will be transferred to the surgical ward. The transition to the ward means the immediate intensive post-operative monitoring of the recovery room is replaced by regular nursing assessments at defined intervals, while you begin the process of settling into what will be your home for the next several days.

Depending on the complexity and duration of your surgery and your baseline health, you may spend the first post-operative night in a high-dependency unit, a step-up care environment with closer monitoring than a standard ward but less intensive than an intensive care unit. This is not a sign that something has gone wrong. For longer, more complex procedures or for patients with significant medical comorbidities, the high-dependency environment is simply the most appropriate place for the first night.

EARLY MOBILISATION — THE MOST IMPORTANT EARLY RECOVERY ACTIVITY

One of the most important things that modern evidence-based post-operative care has established is that early mobilisation, meaning getting up and moving as soon as it is safely possible after surgery, is profoundly beneficial. The era of prolonged post-operative bed rest is over. Studies consistently show that early mobilisation reduces the risk of deep vein thrombosis, reduces the risk of post-operative chest complications including atelectasis and pneumonia, reduces the risk of pressure sores, promotes bowel function recovery, reduces the psychological impact of feeling confined and helpless, and shortens hospital stay.

For most patients undergoing scoliosis surgery, the first mobilisation occurs within 24 hours of surgery, often on the afternoon or evening of the day of operation for morning cases. The physiotherapy team leads this process, providing both the physical assistance and the coaching needed for those first terrifying attempts to sit up and stand.

The technique for getting out of bed after posterior spinal surgery is the log-roll method. Rather than sitting straight up from lying, which would require bending and twisting the recently operated spine, you roll as a single unit onto one side, push up with your arms while your legs swing over the edge of the bed simultaneously, and bring your spine to upright as a rigid unit without bending or twisting. The physiotherapist will teach you this technique and supervise your early attempts.

The first time you stand after major spinal surgery, a combination of post-anaesthetic physiological changes, the effects of remaining medications, and orthostatic hypotension, which is a drop in blood pressure when you transition from lying to standing, can make you feel dizzy or faint. This is normal and is managed by standing slowly in stages, with support, and pausing before attempting to walk. It typically improves rapidly over the first one or two days as your physiology stabilises.

MANAGING PAIN ON THE WARD

Pain management continues as a major focus of care throughout your hospital stay. The principles are consistent with those described for the recovery room: regular baseline medications given around the clock supplemented by patient-controlled or nurse-administered breakthrough doses for uncontrolled pain episodes.

It is important to use your pain medications as directed rather than waiting until pain is severe. Pain is much easier to manage when it is maintained at a baseline level than when it is allowed to build and then requires much larger doses to bring under control. If your pain is not adequately controlled despite taking your medications as prescribed, inform your nursing team. There are almost always additional options that can be tried.

Be aware that opioid medications cause constipation as a side effect. Stool softeners and mild laxatives are prescribed routinely after surgery specifically to manage this. Bowel function typically does not return to normal for two to three days after major surgery, partly due to the opioids and partly due to the physiological response to surgery itself. This is expected and will resolve.

MONITORING AND BLOOD MANAGEMENT

Your vital signs, including blood pressure, heart rate, oxygen saturation, temperature, and respiratory rate, are monitored regularly throughout your hospital stay. The frequency of these checks decreases as your condition stabilises, but they continue throughout your admission.

Daily blood tests in the early post-operative period monitor your haemoglobin level, kidney function, electrolyte balance, and other parameters. A drop in haemoglobin below a threshold considered safe for your individual circumstances, typically around 70 to 80 grams per litre, may prompt a decision to transfuse. Blood transfusion after major scoliosis surgery is not an uncommon occurrence, and you should not be alarmed if it is recommended.

Blood clot prevention is an active part of post-operative care. Deep vein thrombosis, the formation of a clot in the deep veins of the leg, and pulmonary embolism, the migration of such a clot to the lungs, are recognised risks after major surgery. Prevention strategies include early mobilisation, which is the most important single preventive measure, pneumatic sequential compression devices applied to the calves, and in many cases pharmacological anticoagulation started within 24 to 48 hours of surgery.

NUTRITION IN HOSPITAL

Eating and drinking well during the hospital stay supports recovery and should begin as soon as you feel able to manage it. Many patients have minimal appetite in the first day or two after surgery, which is a normal physiological response to major surgical stress. Clear fluids typically begin within hours of surgery, progressing to a light diet and then normal food as appetite and bowel function return.

Prioritise protein-rich foods when you do eat. Hospital catering may not always make it easy to achieve high protein intake, and supplemental protein drinks are often available from the nursing staff or from the hospital pharmacy. Your family can also bring in high-protein foods from outside if this is permitted by the unit's infection control policies.

WOUND CARE AND DRAIN MANAGEMENT

Your surgical wound is closed and covered with a dressing. Wound drains, if placed, typically drain blood-stained fluid in the first 24 to 48 hours, progressively becoming more serous and clear as drainage decreases. Drains are generally removed when output has fallen below a threshold, usually within 48 hours of surgery.

The wound dressing is checked regularly by nursing staff for signs of excessive bleeding or wound problems. You should not attempt to inspect or interfere with the dressing yourself, but you should immediately inform the nursing staff if you notice the dressing becoming saturated with blood, if you develop fever, or if you notice any unusual pain, swelling, or redness around the wound.

FROM THE SURGEON'S DESK

The post-operative period in hospital can feel long or short depending on how things go. For patients with smooth recoveries, the days pass in a pattern of pain management, physiotherapy, meals, and gradually increasing activities, with each day bringing measurable improvement. For patients who encounter a setback, whether a slower recovery of bowel function, a wound issue requiring attention, or an unexpectedly painful night, the ward can feel like a very difficult place.

What I tell every patient before they leave for surgery is that setbacks in the first few days are not the same as the surgery failing. Major scoliosis surgery is physiologically demanding, and recovery is not a uniformly upward line. There will be better days and harder days. The trajectory over weeks is what matters, and for the vast majority of patients, that trajectory is firmly upward.

If something concerns you on the ward, tell the nurses. Do not lie quietly worrying that you are being bothersome. You are there precisely so that any concerns can be attended to, and nursing staff would far rather address a concern that turns out to be normal variation than miss something that needs action.

CHAPTER THIRTEEN:

GOING HOME THE FIRST WEEKS OF RECOVERY

Discharge from hospital is a milestone that most patients eagerly anticipate, and rightly so. It means the acute phase of surgery is behind you, your condition is stable enough to be managed outside the hospital environment, and the next chapter of recovery can begin. But for many patients, going home also marks the moment when the full reality of what they have undergone arrives. The structured support of the hospital, with its round-the-clock nursing presence, ready access to medications, and physiotherapy team on call, is replaced by the reality of home life. That transition demands a great deal more from the patient and their support network than the hospital stay did, and being well-prepared for it makes an enormous difference to how smoothly it goes.

This chapter is a comprehensive guide to the first four to six weeks at home. It covers what to expect day by day, how to manage pain effectively, how to care for the surgical wound, what activities are appropriate at what stage, the emotional dimensions of this period, and when to be concerned and contact your surgical team.

WHAT THE FIRST DAYS AT HOME FEEL LIKE

For most patients, the first several days at home are characterised by significant fatigue, persistent but manageable pain, reduced mobility, and the quieter but no less real challenge of adapting to a temporarily different version of daily life. Understanding that this is normal, and that it does not indicate a problem with your recovery, is one of the most important things this chapter can offer you.

Fatigue after major surgery runs deeper than ordinary tiredness and can surprise patients who expected to feel meaningfully better once they were home. The body is conducting an enormous amount of biological work in the weeks after major surgery: managing the inflammatory response, healing the surgical wound, beginning the long process of bone fusion across the operated segments, and maintaining all the normal physiological demands of life simultaneously. This biological labour consumes energy that would otherwise be available for activity and alertness. The fatigue you feel is appropriate and real, and resting is not laziness. It is an active component of recovery.

A useful practical framework for the early days at home is the activity-rest cycle. Plan short periods of gentle activity, which in the first week means little more than walking around the house or a short distance outside, followed by periods of rest of similar or greater length. As the days and weeks pass, gradually extend the activity periods and reduce the rest periods in proportion to your improving stamina and reducing pain.

Sleep in the early weeks at home is frequently disrupted by pain, by the challenge of finding and maintaining comfortable positions in bed, by the physiological effects of post-operative medications, and by the anxiety that naturally accompanies a period of major physical vulnerability. Many patients find sleeping in a semi-reclined position, in a recliner chair or propped up with multiple pillows, more comfortable than lying fully flat in the first week or two. The semi-reclined position reduces loading on the lumbar spine and is often easier to get into and out of than a flat bed position. Experiment with what works best for your own body.

PAIN MANAGEMENT AT HOME IN DETAIL

Leaving hospital does not mean leaving pain management behind. You will be discharged with prescriptions for analgesic medications covering the weeks ahead. These typically include paracetamol for baseline analgesia, an opioid medication such as tramadol, codeine, or oxycodone for breakthrough pain, and potentially a nerve-modulating agent such as pregabalin or gabapentin if this was part of your inpatient regimen.

The single most important principle of home pain management is to take medications on a schedule rather than waiting until pain is severe. Analgesics work far more effectively when they maintain a steady therapeutic level in the bloodstream than when they are taken reactively after pain has built to a peak. Take your regular medications at the prescribed times whether or not pain is currently intense, and use your breakthrough medication at the first sign of escalating pain rather than attempting to tolerate it while it worsens.

Track your pain and medication use in a simple daily diary. Record your pain score on a zero to ten scale at consistent times each day alongside what medications you took and when. This objective record is valuable at follow-up appointments because it provides accurate data about your progress rather than a general impression coloured by a particularly difficult or surprisingly good recent day.

Managing opioid medications at home requires specific awareness. These medications are necessary and effective for post-surgical pain, but they require careful use. Constipation is almost universal with opioid use and must be managed from the first day home with stool softeners taken daily, progressing to stimulant laxatives if needed. Do not drive, operate machinery, or make important decisions while taking opioid analgesics. Do not consume alcohol alongside them. Monitor your own requirements with the goal of progressively reducing opioid use as pain allows, as dependency can develop with prolonged unmonitored use.

If after two to three weeks your opioid requirements are not decreasing, or if you find yourself using breakthrough medication many times daily on a persistent basis, discuss this with your surgical team. There are almost always additional strategies available, and your team wants to know if pain is not adequately controlled.

Non-pharmacological approaches to pain complement medications and are worth incorporating consistently. Cold packs or ice wrapped in a cloth applied to the wound area for 15 to 20 minutes at a time several times daily can meaningfully reduce local inflammatory pain. Careful positioning with pillow support to maintain the spine in a comfortable, neutral alignment reduces background discomfort during rest. Gentle walking, as described below, reduces muscle stiffness and promotes the circulation that supports healing. Distraction through engaging activities, reading, conversations, podcasts, and television, reduces pain perception by redirecting attentional resources.

WOUND CARE — KEEPING THE HEALING PROCESS SAFE

Your surgical wound at discharge will be covered with a dressing and you will have been given specific instructions about its management. Follow these instructions carefully rather than improvising, as wound care protocols reflect evidence about what promotes healing and reduces infection risk.

The fundamental principles are consistent. Keep the wound clean and dry. Do not immerse the wound in water, meaning no baths, no swimming, no soaking, until the wound is fully healed and you have explicit clearance from your surgical team. Showering is generally permitted from the first or second day after discharge, usually with the dressing in place or with a waterproof cover, but check your specific instructions. After showering, gently pat the wound area dry rather than rubbing across it.

Change the dressing according to your schedule, typically every two to three days or when it becomes saturated, visibly soiled, or begins to lift at the edges. Always wash your hands thoroughly before any dressing change. At each change, carefully observe the wound for signs of normal healing progression and for any warning signs of problems.

Normal healing signs include a clean wound line with no gaping, some redness and warmth in the first week that gradually diminishes, and minimal clear or slightly straw-coloured fluid if drainage is present. Warning signs that require contact with your surgical team include redness spreading around the wound edges that is increasing rather than decreasing after the first week, warmth of the wound area that is increasing, swelling that is growing, discharge from the wound that is opaque, thick, greenish, or has an unpleasant odour, and any fever defined as a temperature above 38 degrees Celsius. These signs may indicate infection, which is best treated when identified early.

External sutures or staples are removed at approximately 10 to 14 days, either at your first post-operative clinic appointment or by a community nurse. After their removal, the wound continues to heal internally and the scar matures over the following months. The scar may remain firm, raised, and tender for several months before softening and flattening. Silicone gel strips or silicone scar sheets applied once the wound is fully closed can help improve the long-term appearance of the scar and are available without prescription.

THE ACTIVITY PROGRAMME — PROGRESSIVE AND GUIDED

Managing activity in the early weeks requires balancing the need to move enough to prevent complications and support recovery against the need to protect the healing surgical site from excessive load. The specific guidance you receive from your surgical and physiotherapy team will reflect your individual procedure and recovery, and should always take precedence over the general guidance here.

Walking is the foundational activity of early recovery and its importance cannot be overstated. From the first day home, walk around the house. Each subsequent day, aim to walk a little further. By the end of the first week, most patients can manage a short walk outside on flat terrain. By the end of the second week, the target is 10 to 15 minutes of continuous walking. By weeks four to six, 20 to 30 minutes twice daily is a realistic goal for most patients with uncomplicated recoveries.

Walking is safe for the recovering fusion. The gentle compressive loading it generates is within the tolerance of a well-instrumented spinal construct. It improves cardiovascular conditioning, dramatically reduces the risk of deep vein thrombosis, promotes bowel function, reduces paraspinal muscle stiffness, and is one of the most evidence-based mood-improving activities available.

Activities to avoid in the first six weeks are those generating excessive spinal load, torsional force, or fall risk. Do not lift anything heavier than approximately two to three kilograms, which is roughly the weight of a full kettle or a small bag of groceries. Do not bend forward at the waist. Do not twist the spine. Do not run, jump, or participate in any sport. Limit sitting to short periods initially, as sustained sitting generates significant lumbar loading. When you must sit, choose a firm chair at a height that allows you to sit with hips and knees at approximately 90 degrees, and rise by pushing up with your arms rather than bending the trunk forward.

THE EMOTIONAL LANDSCAPE OF EARLY RECOVERY

Recovery from major surgery is a psychological journey as much as a physical one. The emotional experience of the first weeks at home is genuinely complex, and patients are better prepared to navigate it when they understand in advance that it will be.

Post-surgical emotional dip is a recognised and nearly universal phenomenon affecting patients in the first two to four weeks after major surgery. It encompasses low mood, periods of tearfulness, irritability, anxiety, and a general sense of vulnerability that is difficult to articulate but real and common. Its sources are multiple and interacting: the physiological stress response to major surgery, the effects of opioid medications which can cause dysphoria in some individuals, disrupted sleep, reduced autonomy and independence, the replacement of the busy purposeful focus of pre-operative preparation with the slower, more passive work of recovery, and the simple difficulty of daily life being temporarily harder than it was before.

This emotional dip is not clinical depression in most cases, and it typically resolves naturally and progressively as pain decreases, function improves, and the milestones of recovery begin to accumulate. Each small achievement, the first walk to the end of the road, the first night of adequate sleep, the first day without needing the strongest medications, contributes to a gradually rebuilding sense of progress and capability.

Strategies that help during this period include maintaining human connection. Social interaction, whether in person, by phone, or video call, is one of the most powerful antidotes to the isolation that restricted mobility can produce. Set small, achievable daily goals and acknowledge when you meet them. Keep a simple recovery journal, noting progress rather than only difficulties. Engage in activities that provide mental stimulation and enjoyment within the physical constraints of this period: reading, listening to audiobooks or podcasts, creative activities, learning something new.

If emotional difficulty feels severe, is not improving, or feels like it is getting worse as the weeks pass rather than better, discuss it with your surgical team or general practitioner. Targeted psychological support during recovery is available and effective, and accessing it is not a sign of failure. It is a sign of intelligent self-care.

FROM THE SURGEON'S DESK

The question I am most consistently asked by patients at discharge is: how will I know if something is wrong?

The answer I give covers the specific warning signs that require prompt contact with the surgical team or, if they are unreachable, with emergency services. Worsening pain representing a significant change from the recent trend, particularly if not responding to prescribed medications. Any new or worsening neurological symptoms: new weakness in legs or feet, new numbness or tingling, any change in bladder or bowel control. These require urgent assessment without delay. Signs of wound infection as described above. Fever above 38 degrees Celsius. Swelling, warmth, or redness in one or both calves that could represent deep vein thrombosis. Chest pain or shortness of breath, which requires emergency assessment.

None of these are common. Most patients go home and recover without encountering any of them. But knowing them means that if they do occur, you will recognise them and act promptly. In the rare situations where complications arise, the speed of recognition and response is one of the most important determinants of outcome.

CHAPTER FOURTEEN:

REHABILITATION AND GETTING BACK TO LIFE

Recovery from scoliosis surgery is not a passive process that unfolds automatically over time without effort or engagement. It is an active, structured journey that requires consistent commitment from the patient, skilled guidance from the physiotherapy and surgical teams, and the patience to work within a timeline that is determined by biology rather than desire. The surgery corrects the structural problem. Rehabilitation restores function, strength, and confidence. Both are essential, and neither can substitute for the other.

This chapter covers the full arc of rehabilitation from the early weeks at home through the months of progressive recovery, the milestones to expect at different stages, the return to sport and full physical activity, and the longer-term relationship with a fused spine.

THE THREE PHASES OF REHABILITATION

Rehabilitation after scoliosis surgery is most clearly understood as a three-phase process. The phases overlap rather than following sharp boundaries, and the progression between them is guided by clinical assessment and imaging rather than by the calendar alone. Understanding these phases gives you a framework for interpreting the guidance you receive and for managing your expectations about the pace of change.

Phase One: Protection and Early Restoration (Weeks One to Six)

The overarching goal of phase one is to protect the surgical site from loads that could compromise the instrumentation or the early fusion biology, while simultaneously beginning the early restoration of mobility, circulation, and basic daily function. The bone fusion at this stage is in its earliest biological phase: cellular ingrowth has begun and early bone matrix is being deposited, but the construct has no structural independence from the metal instrumentation. The implants are bearing the full mechanical load.

The walking programme is the defining activity of phase one and is described in detail in Chapter Thirteen. It is safe, beneficial, and should be the primary physical focus. Progressive daily increases in walking distance and duration drive the most important early recovery gains.

Breathing exercises are an important component of phase one, particularly after thoracic surgery where the rib cage has been in proximity to the surgical field. Deep breathing exercises using the full thoracic and abdominal excursion of the respiratory system prevent atelectasis, maintain respiratory muscle function, and promote the full expansion of the lungs. These exercises take only a few minutes but should be performed several times daily.

Early physiotherapy sessions in this phase focus primarily on education and safety confirmation. The physiotherapist assesses your movement patterns, confirms that your log-roll technique is correct and safe, identifies any compensatory patterns that might cause problems, ensures your home exercise programme is being performed correctly, and monitors your progress against expected milestones.

By the end of phase one, most patients with uncomplicated recoveries can walk 20 to 30 minutes continuously, manage personal care independently, manage stairs safely, ride in a car for short journeys, and begin sedentary work or study if this is their occupation.

Phase Two: Strengthening and Functional Expansion (Weeks Six to Sixteen)

As fusion matures and pain progressively reduces, the rehabilitation programme expands significantly in both scope and intensity. The biological situation has evolved: bone bridging across the fused segments is becoming more established, the instrumentation is sharing load with the developing bony union, and the spine is increasingly capable of tolerating greater mechanical demands.

Core stabilisation is the central focus of phase two physiotherapy. The deep stabilising muscles of the trunk, specifically the transversus abdominis, multifidus, and pelvic floor muscles, form the inner muscular corset that provides dynamic stabilisation to the lumbar spine during movement. These muscles are frequently inhibited in the post-operative period due to pain, surgical disruption, and the protective muscular guarding response. Their re-activation and progressive strengthening is a major rehabilitation goal because it directly supports the developing fusion and reduces long-term back pain risk.

It is important to clarify what core strengthening in this context means. It does not mean the aggressive, high-load core exercises of general fitness training: crunches, sit-ups, heavy planks, or loaded rotational exercises are inappropriate in the first several months after spinal fusion. Phase two core exercises are gentle, controlled activation exercises that specifically target the deep stabilisers in neutral spine positions, without generating significant compressive or shear loading of the fusion. Your physiotherapist will teach these specifically.

Flexibility work becomes an important phase two component as pain reduction permits. The hip flexors and iliopsoas muscles, the hamstrings, the thoracic rotators, and the shoulder girdle muscles all tend to become shortened and tight during the restricted movement of the recovery period. Regular, sustained stretching of these structures improves posture, reduces muscular back pain, and prepares the body for the expanded activities of later recovery phases.

Swimming in a formal, supervised setting is an excellent phase two activity. The buoyancy of water reduces spinal loading substantially while allowing a wide range of controlled movement, making it one of the safest and most beneficial rehabilitation activities for recovering spinal fusion patients. Most surgeons clear supervised swimming at approximately 10 to 12 weeks post-operatively. The initial sessions should be gentle laps at a comfortable pace, avoiding strokes that generate significant spinal rotation such as breaststroke, and building progressively.

Stationary cycling provides cardiovascular conditioning without impact and is generally appropriate from eight to twelve weeks. The controlled, repetitive motion of cycling does not generate problematic spinal loading and is well-tolerated by most patients in this recovery phase.

Phase Three: Return to Full Activity (Months Four to Twelve and Beyond)

The transition into phase three is marked by imaging evidence of advancing fusion, clinical assessment confirming adequate spinal stability, and the patient's own sense of readily tolerating the expanded demands of phase two. By four to six months in most uncomplicated cases, patients are ready to progressively challenge themselves toward full return to activity.

Phase three rehabilitation involves progressively more demanding exercise including light gym-based resistance training building core and global muscle strength, more challenging cardiovascular activities, and the structured reintroduction of sport under guidance. Resistance exercises at this stage must be carefully selected to avoid excessive loading of the fused segments, and the progression should be guided by your physiotherapist in communication with your surgical team.

The specific timelines for return to individual activities vary considerably. Light recreational exercise, moderate cycling, recreational swimming, and social activities without significant physical demand are typically possible by months four to six. Progressive return to sport, including recreational running on flat surfaces, doubles tennis, golf, and recreational skiing, typically follows between months six and nine. Contact sport, heavy weightlifting, competitive athletics, gymnastics, and martial arts require a minimum of twelve months and explicit surgical clearance.

RETURN TO SPORT — THE EVIDENCE

The evidence on return to sport after scoliosis surgery is overall encouraging and important for patients and families with sporting aspirations to understand clearly rather than allowing anxiety to replace data.

Multiple published studies following cohorts of active patients after adolescent idiopathic scoliosis surgery have documented return-to-sport rates of 80 to 95 percent at one to two years, with the large majority returning to their pre-operative level of activity. Studies specifically examining competitive athletes have found that high-level sporting performance, including competitive swimming, athletics, and team sports, is achievable after scoliosis fusion with appropriate rehabilitation and timing.

Dance, including pre-professional and professional ballet and contemporary dance, has been specifically studied. Published evidence demonstrates that dancers can return to professional-level performance after scoliosis surgery, though the timeline is extended relative to recreational sport, typically 12 to 18 months to full dance training, with a carefully graduated return programme developed in collaboration between the surgical team and the patient's dance teacher.

High-impact, high-load activities including competitive gymnastics, heavyweight lifting, and American football lineman positions, where very high axial compressive loads are generated repeatedly, require specific discussion with the surgical team about risks and realistic expectations given the specific extent of fusion in each patient's case.

OCCUPATIONAL REHABILITATION

Return to work and educational commitments is a significant rehabilitation milestone for most patients. The appropriate timeline depends fundamentally on the physical demands of the specific occupation or academic environment.

Sedentary work involving primarily sitting, computer use, or light administrative tasks can generally be considered at four to six weeks, initially part-time, progressing to full-time over the following weeks as stamina allows. Many patients in sedentary roles find a graduated return, three to four hours daily initially increasing by an hour or two each week, more manageable than a sudden full return.

Driving-dependent work must wait until driving is cleared by the surgeon, typically at six to eight weeks for most patients. The specific driving restrictions relate to both the medications being taken and the physical demands of driving.

Manual labour, nursing, teaching with significant standing and moving demands, construction, and any work involving lifting or sustained physical effort typically requires three to six months minimum. For heavy manual occupations, this timeline may extend to six to twelve months. An occupational health assessment through your employer, with a formal graduated return-to-work plan, is appropriate for physically demanding occupations.

THE LONG-TERM RELATIONSHIP WITH YOUR SPINE

One of the most important messages for patients completing their rehabilitation is that the goal of scoliosis surgery was never to create a spine that needs to be protected from life. It was to create a spine capable of supporting full participation in life. The evidence from long-term outcome studies strongly supports this message.

Patients who maintain active, physically engaged lifestyles after scoliosis surgery have consistently better outcomes than those who become sedentary: better pain scores, better function, better psychological wellbeing, and better overall quality of life. Regular physical activity maintains the health of the disc and facet joints in the unfused segments adjacent to the fusion, reduces the rate of adjacent segment degeneration, supports body weight management that reduces spinal loading, and is one of the most powerful contributors to long-term physical and psychological health.

The practical recommendation is specific. Once cleared by your surgeon, aim for at least 150 minutes of moderate-intensity cardiovascular activity weekly, build and maintain core strength through regular specific exercises, maintain general muscle strength and flexibility through a balanced exercise programme, and listen to your body with intelligent attention rather than fearful restriction.

FROM THE SURGEON'S DESK

I follow patients for years after surgery. The range of lives they return to never fails to move me. Runners. Swimmers. Skiers. Rock climbers. Dancers. Footballers. Parents chasing toddlers. Workers in physically demanding trades. Travellers who carry their own bags.

Not every patient achieves every aspiration, and I would be dishonest to promise that. Individual outcomes depend on the extent of surgery, the age at operation, the quality of rehabilitation, and the biological variables of healing that we cannot fully control. But what the long-term evidence consistently shows, and what I see reflected in my own patients' lives, is that the potential for full and active participation in life after well-performed scoliosis surgery is real, evidence-based, and should be the expected outcome rather than the hoped-for exception.

The patients who achieve the best long-term outcomes are not necessarily those with the most anatomically favourable situations. They are the ones who engage fully with rehabilitation, who respect the timeline while pushing themselves appropriately within it, and who refuse to let the fact of having had surgery become a ceiling on what they believe they are capable of.

Part Five

Risks, Complications And Long-Term Outcomes

CHAPTER FIFTEEN:

RISKS, COMPLICATIONS, AND HONEST ANSWERS

Informed consent is a cornerstone of ethical surgical practice. Before you agree to any procedure, you are entitled to complete and comprehensible information about its purpose, expected benefits, risks, and available alternatives. This chapter honours that requirement by providing a thorough, honest, and clinically accurate account of the risks of scoliosis surgery, how those risks are managed, and how to think about them clearly.

HOW TO THINK ABOUT SURGICAL RISK

Absolute versus relative risk is an important distinction for understanding risk information. An absolute risk is a direct probability: a one percent risk means one patient in every 100 experiences that outcome. Ninety-nine do not. A relative risk compares groups: smokers have twice the non-union risk of non-smokers. That relative figure sounds alarming, but if the baseline non-union rate is two percent, doubling it produces four percent, which remains a minority outcome. Always seek absolute rather than relative risk figures.

The comparison to untreated disease is the essential context for every surgical risk. The risks of scoliosis surgery must always be weighed against the risks of the untreated condition: progressive curve, worsening pain, functional decline, and in severe thoracic curves, cardiorespiratory compromise over decades. For most patients being advised that surgery is appropriate, this comparison is what ultimately makes the risk-benefit balance clear.

Surgeon and institution experience substantially modifies risk. Complication rates at high-volume specialist centres are consistently and substantially lower than those reported from lower-volume settings across virtually every category of complication. This is one of the most important reasons to ensure that major scoliosis surgery is performed by an experienced specialist team.

NEUROLOGICAL INJURY — THE MOST FEARED RISK

Neurological injury, damage to the spinal cord or nerve roots causing weakness, paralysis, numbness, or loss of bladder and bowel control, is the complication that most patients fear most. Understanding the actual risk in contemporary practice is essential for an accurate rather than catastrophised perception of the procedure.

In adolescent idiopathic scoliosis surgery at specialist centres with continuous intraoperative neurophysiological monitoring, the risk of significant permanent neurological deficit is approximately 0.5 to 1 percent in published large series. Expressed differently, 99 to 99.5 percent of patients do not experience permanent neurological injury. In the highest-volume specialist centres with consistent monitoring, this rate is lower still.

The continuous use of IONM throughout the procedure is the primary safety intervention for neurological complications. When monitoring detects a signal change indicating possible compromise of spinal cord or nerve root function, the surgical team responds immediately: releasing corrective forces, checking implant positions, adjusting the surgical plan, or administering pharmacological agents to support spinal cord perfusion. This response capability is why early detection through monitoring is so valuable: a transient change detected and corrected is not a complication. It is the monitoring system doing precisely what it was designed to do.

SURGICAL SITE INFECTION

Deep wound infection after scoliosis surgery occurs in approximately one to four percent of cases. The rate varies with patient factors including diabetes, obesity, smoking, immunosuppression, and nutritional deficiency, and with surgical factors including operative duration and blood loss.

Superficial infections confined to the skin and subcutaneous tissues are managed with antibiotics and wound care and typically resolve completely. Deep infections involving the fascial layers or the implants are more serious and may require surgical washout under anaesthesia. In severe or refractory deep infections, staged management including temporary implant removal may be necessary.

Prevention includes pre-operative antiseptic skin preparation, prophylactic antibiotics given before skin incision and continued post-operatively per protocol, careful intraoperative tissue handling, and meticulous wound closure. Patients can contribute to infection prevention by optimising nutritional status, stopping smoking, managing diabetes carefully, and following all wound care instructions after discharge.

BLOOD LOSS AND TRANSFUSION MANAGEMENT

Significant blood loss accompanies major scoliosis surgery, and managing this safely is a major component of perioperative care. For a standard posterior adolescent idiopathic scoliosis fusion, blood loss in the range of 500 to 1500 millilitres is typical. Adult deformity procedures involving osteotomies may involve substantially greater losses.

Intraoperative cell salvage collects, processes, and returns the patient's own shed blood throughout the procedure, recovering a substantial proportion of losses as transfusable autologous blood. This is the most effective blood conservation technique and is standard practice at experienced centres. Tranexamic acid, a medication that inhibits fibrinolysis, is given routinely before and during surgery to reduce total blood loss. Controlled hypotensive anaesthesia reduces blood loss by maintaining blood pressure at the lower end of the safe range during surgery.

Despite these measures, blood transfusion is required in some patients and is not itself a complication. Blood is carefully cross-matched, screened, and administered according to strict clinical protocols.

IMPLANT-RELATED COMPLICATIONS

Screw malposition means a pedicle screw placed outside its intended position within the pedicle and vertebral body. Most minor malpositions identified on post-operative imaging are clinically inconsequential. Significant malpositions that encroach on neural structures or compromise fixation may require revision. Navigation-guided screw placement significantly reduces malposition rates compared to conventional freehand technique.

Rod fracture occurs at a stress concentration point in the rod, typically years after surgery in patients where the fusion has not fully matured. It presents with new localised back pain and is confirmed on imaging. Management is individualised based on symptoms, the degree of fusion at adjacent levels, and the overall clinical picture.

Adjacent segment disease means accelerated degenerative changes developing in the spinal levels immediately above or below the fused construct, related to the increased mechanical demands placed on these mobile segments by the immobile fusion. The risk is higher in adult patients whose adjacent segments may already show degenerative changes. Symptomatic adjacent segment disease requiring surgical management occurs in a minority of patients over long-term follow-up.

NON-UNION — FAILURE OF FUSION

Pseudarthrosis, or non-union, means that bone graft has failed to form a solid bony bridge across one or more segments of the fusion, leaving those segments without biological support for the instrumentation. Unrecognised and untreated non-union leads to progressive implant fatigue and eventual failure.

Risk factors are clearly identified: smoking is the most powerful modifiable risk factor, dramatically increasing non-union rates through its adverse effects on bone cell function and local blood supply. Diabetes, osteoporosis, nutritional deficiency, and very long fusion constructs also increase risk.

Treatment of identified non-union involves revision surgery to refresh the fusion bed, augment fixation, and add additional bone graft with biological adjuncts. Revision procedures for pseudarthrosis achieve solid fusion in the majority of cases.

DURAL TEAR AND CSF LEAK

Inadvertent entry through the dura mater during surgical dissection occurs in approximately one to five percent of primary scoliosis procedures, with higher rates in revision surgery where scar tissue complicates dissection. When identified intraoperatively, the dural tear is repaired with fine suture and sealant. Post-operatively, the patient may need to lie flat for a period while the repair heals, and may experience positional headaches from reduced cerebrospinal fluid pressure when upright. The large majority resolve completely without permanent neurological consequences.

FROM THE SURGEON'S DESK

When I go through risks with patients, I try to give an accurate picture rather than either minimising them with false reassurance or presenting them in a way that generates disproportionate fear. Honest risk communication serves patients far better than either extreme.

The honest picture is this: serious complications occur in a minority of patients undergoing scoliosis surgery at specialist centres. The most feared complication, permanent neurological injury, is uncommon in experienced hands with full intraoperative monitoring. The surgical community has worked intensively for decades to reduce these rates, and contemporary complication data reflect that sustained effort.

But risk cannot be reduced to zero, and patients deserve to know that. The appropriate response to this reality is not to avoid surgery when it is genuinely indicated. It is to ensure that the procedure is performed by the most experienced team available, at a centre with the infrastructure and expertise to manage the full range of potential complications effectively if they arise.

CHAPTER SIXTEEN:

REVISION SURGERY WHEN A SECOND OPERATION IS NEEDED

Revision surgery, a second or subsequent spinal procedure to address a problem arising from or following the first, is one of the most difficult conversations in scoliosis care. No patient wants to hear it is necessary, and the emotional response, a combination of disappointment, frustration, fear, and sometimes anger, is entirely understandable and legitimate. This chapter gives patients and families facing this possibility a clear, honest understanding of what revision surgery is, why it is needed, what it involves, and what outcomes can realistically be expected.

WHAT REVISION SURGERY MEANS — AND WHAT IT DOES NOT

Revision surgery in scoliosis is not equivalent to a procedure that failed in the meaningful sense. It is not, in most cases, the correction of a surgical error. It is the management of a recognised complication or the natural progression of complex biological processes in a patient whose primary surgery was performed appropriately, but whose healing, mechanical situation, or adjacent anatomy has evolved in a way requiring further surgical attention.

This distinction matters profoundly for patients emotionally. Being told you need revision surgery can feel like learning that the initial operation let you down. In the majority of cases, that is not an accurate reading of the situation. The biology of bone healing is imperfect and variable between patients. The mechanical environment of a long spinal construct under years of cyclical loading is demanding. Adjacent segments may develop changes requiring management that cannot be predicted at the time of primary surgery. These are features of a complex biological process, not surgical failures.

INDICATIONS FOR REVISION SURGERY

Implant-related failure encompasses problems with the hardware placed at primary surgery. Rod fracture presents with new localised back pain at the fracture level, sometimes with a palpable change in the back contour, and is confirmed by imaging. Management is individualised: a fracture in a solidly fused construct with minimal symptoms may be observed; one associated with pain, progressive deformity, or pseudarthrosis at that level typically requires revision with rod replacement and additional bone graft augmentation. Screw loosening or pullout, most commonly seen in osteoporotic patients or those who have not achieved solid fusion, may require revision with augmented fixation techniques including cement augmentation to increase screw purchase in compromised bone.

Pseudarthrosis requiring revision presents with localised back pain, sometimes associated with radiographic evidence of motion at the non-union level or fracture of the implants. The revision procedure involves re-exposing the affected levels, thoroughly preparing the failed fusion bed by removing fibrous tissue and exposing fresh bleeding cancellous bone surfaces, augmenting fixation as needed, and adding bone graft supplemented with biological adjuncts such as BMP to maximise fusion biology at the revision.

Junctional failure requiring revision refers to proximal or distal junctional kyphosis that has progressed to a severity causing significant pain, neurological compromise, or substantial loss of correction. Mild junctional kyphosis is common and frequently asymptomatic, requiring observation rather than intervention. Severe junctional failure with clinical consequences typically requires extension of the fusion to include the affected adjacent levels.

Neurological complications requiring prompt revision include post-operative haematoma compressing the neural structures, which presents with rapidly progressive neurological deficit and requires emergency surgical evacuation, and implant malposition causing nerve root or spinal cord compression, which may require repositioning or removal of the offending implant.

THE TECHNICAL CHALLENGES OF REVISION

Revision scoliosis surgery is unambiguously more technically demanding than primary surgery in virtually every dimension. Surgeons who perform revision cases regularly understand and are prepared for these challenges. Surgeons who do not perform them regularly are not the appropriate choice for revision procedures.

Scar tissue from the previous operation obliterates the normal tissue planes that guide dissection in primary surgery. Structures that can be cleanly and safely identified in a virgin field are adherent to fibrotic scar and require more cautious, methodical dissection to identify and protect. Operating time is correspondingly longer.

Existing implants embedded in varying degrees of bone ingrowth and fibrous tissue require careful removal. The bone at the interface with removed implants may be damaged or deficient, requiring specific strategies for creating new fixation points in compromised anatomy.

The requirement for revision surgery underscores once again why the initial procedure should be performed at a specialist centre with experience in the full spectrum of scoliosis management, including revision cases, because the experience of managing complex primary cases is the foundation on which revision expertise is built.

EMOTIONAL SUPPORT THROUGH REVISION

The emotional experience of revision surgery deserves explicit acknowledgment and support rather than clinical bypassing in the rush to discuss the surgical plan.

Many patients describe a sense of having endured everything the first surgery asked of them, rebuilt their lives, returned to function, and then been told they must begin again. This experience can evoke genuine grief, and approaching it as such rather than purely as a technical problem to be solved is part of caring for the whole person.

Several realities are genuinely available as sources of comfort. Revision surgery for the most common indications, including pseudarthrosis, rod fracture, and junctional failure, achieves good clinical outcomes in the majority of cases. Patients who have already navigated one major scoliosis surgery and recovery have demonstrated a capacity for this that has genuine value. They know more about what to expect. They have existing relationships with their surgical team. They have already proven to themselves that they can do this.

FROM THE SURGEON'S DESK

Telling a patient they need revision surgery is one of the hardest conversations I have. There is no way to soften the news to the point where it does not land hard, and I have stopped trying to. What I try to do instead is have the conversation fully, honestly, and unhurriedly.

I explain exactly what has happened mechanically or biologically, in terms the patient can understand without medical training. I explain what the revision will involve and what we expect to achieve. And I acknowledge the difficulty of the news directly before moving into the clinical discussion, because patients need a moment to absorb what they have heard before they can engage with information about the path forward.

The patients who navigate revision surgery most successfully are those who allow themselves to feel the disappointment and then redirect their considerable demonstrated resilience toward what needs to be done next. They have done this before. They can do it again. And the evidence supports that revision surgery, when clearly indicated and well-performed, gives them the durable outcome they deserve.

CHAPTER SEVENTEEN:

THE PSYCHOLOGICAL AND EMOTIONAL IMPACT OF SCOLIOSIS SURGERY

Scoliosis is more than a spinal condition. For many patients, particularly those who have lived with visible deformity through years of adolescence and young adulthood, it is a psychological and social experience as much as a physical one. Surgery, when successful, has a transformative impact that extends far beyond the radiographic correction visible on X-ray. This chapter explores the psychological dimensions of living with scoliosis, navigating the surgical process, and building a life after surgery.

THE PSYCHOLOGICAL BURDEN OF LIVING WITH SCOLIOSIS

The impact of scoliosis on psychological wellbeing has been carefully studied using validated quality of life instruments, and the findings are consistent and clinically important. Patients with moderate to severe scoliosis score significantly lower on measures of body image, self-concept, social participation, and mental health than age-matched peers without the condition. These are not trivial differences. They represent a real and meaningful diminishment of quality of life occurring across the domains of daily experience, recreational activity, and psychological wellbeing.

Body image is the domain most consistently and profoundly affected. Visible spinal deformity including asymmetric shoulder height, a rib hump visible through clothing, an asymmetric waist, or a prominent hip, shapes how a person sees themselves and how they feel others see them. For adolescents navigating the intense self-consciousness and social evaluation of puberty and early adulthood, these physical differences can feel enormously significant.

Research has documented that adolescents with moderate to severe scoliosis engage in systematic avoidance behaviours: avoiding swimming, sports, and other activities where the body is visible, avoiding close physical contact with peers, and deliberately wearing specific clothing designed to conceal the deformity. These avoidance behaviours compound the social isolation that physical difference can produce and reduce participation in the activities that contribute most to adolescent wellbeing and development.

Adults with progressive degenerative scoliosis carry a different but equally real burden. The gradual loss of function, the progressive intrusion of pain into daily life, the inability to participate in activities previously enjoyed, and in severe cases the loss of normal upright posture and independent ambulation, are profoundly demoralising in ways that the clinical literature on physical outcomes often understates.

THE SURGICAL TRANSFORMATION — BODY IMAGE AND BEYOND

For patients who achieve a good surgical outcome, the psychological impact of surgery can be profound and is consistently among the most meaningful benefits reported by patients themselves. This is documented in the validated self-image domain of the Scoliosis Research Society outcome instrument, which shows significant and sustained improvement after successful surgical correction across studies with follow-up periods of five, ten, and twenty-plus years.

What patients describe in their own words goes beyond clinical measures. They describe standing differently and carrying themselves differently. They describe inhabiting their bodies in a fundamentally changed way. They describe wearing clothes they had avoided for years, participating in activities from which they had excluded themselves, and feeling the reduction of the constant background awareness of physical difference that had shaped their daily experience for as long as they could remember.

Many patients describe the cosmetic improvement of surgery as among its most meaningful benefits, sometimes more meaningful in their daily experience than the pain relief or functional improvement, though these are all deeply interrelated. This is entirely legitimate. The psychological experience of the body is inseparable from the physical experience of it, and surgical correction that addresses the visible dimensions of the deformity along with its structural ones restores something profound to the patient's relationship with their own body and their sense of themselves in the world.

THE EMOTIONAL ARC OF THE SURGICAL JOURNEY

The emotional experience of the surgical journey has a characteristic shape, and understanding this shape in advance helps patients navigate it more effectively.

The pre-operative period is characterised for most patients by a combination of relief that the decision has been made and anxiety about the operation itself. This combination, relief and anxiety existing simultaneously, can be disorienting, and patients may wonder why they do not feel simply resolved now that the path forward is clear. The answer is that both feelings are appropriate and normal. Having the right information, including the detailed content of a book like this one, is the most effective tool for managing the anxiety component.

The peri-operative period, the day of surgery and immediate aftermath, is often described retrospectively as less frightening in reality than it was in anticipation. The combination of being well-prepared, being surrounded by a professional team wholly focused on your care, and the fact that general anaesthesia removes all awareness of the procedure itself means that many patients find the actual surgical day more manageable than the preceding weeks of anticipation.

The early recovery period is frequently the most emotionally challenging phase. The post-surgical emotional dip described in Chapter Thirteen, encompassing low mood, vulnerability, reduced autonomy, and the difficulty of pain-limited daily life, requires acknowledgment and active coping strategies. The patients who navigate it most effectively are those who were prepared for it in advance and who understand it as a normal and temporary feature of recovery rather than a sign that something is wrong.

The later recovery and rehabilitation phase is for most patients a period of progressively building momentum, each milestone of recovery feeding the next in a positive cycle of improving function and mood. By three to six months, most patients with smooth recoveries are experiencing meaningfully improved quality of life compared to their pre-operative state, and this experience of improvement is itself a powerful psychological reward.

PSYCHOLOGICAL SUPPORT IN THE SURGICAL PROCESS

Several levels of psychological support are appropriate and beneficial at different stages of the surgical journey.

Psychological preparation through information and education, represented by this book, is the foundational level. Patients who understand what to expect are less frightened by the experience, more capable of engaging effectively with their recovery, and report better overall satisfaction with the surgical process.

Mindfulness-based practices, as described in Chapter Seven, have genuine evidence behind them for reducing pre-operative anxiety and post-operative pain. They are accessible, free, and can be learned through widely available apps and online resources.

Peer support, through conversations with other patients who have undergone similar procedures, either in person, through hospital programmes, or via reputable online communities, provides both practical information and a form of emotional solidarity that professional support cannot fully replicate.

Clinical psychological support from a psychologist or counsellor experienced in chronic illness and surgical recovery is appropriate and beneficial for patients who are struggling significantly, who have significant pre-existing anxiety or depression, or who have a history of difficult medical experiences. Accessing this support is not a sign of unusual fragility. It is a rational response to a genuinely demanding experience and one that evidence supports as improving clinical outcomes.

FROM THE SURGEON'S DESK

I have been changed by the patients I have operated on. Not in a single dramatic way but in the accumulated effect of years of watching people come through one of the more significant experiences of their lives, and emerge, most of them, with something genuinely transformed.

I operated on a young woman some years ago who had lived with a large thoracic curve since early adolescence. By the time she came to me in her mid-twenties, she had not worn a swimming costume in seven years. She described her scoliosis as a constant presence in every social situation she navigated, an invisible companion that shaped every decision about clothing, activity, and proximity to others. At her one-year follow-up, she showed me photographs from a beach holiday where she had swum in the sea every single day.

That transformation, from hiding to living, from organising daily life around a deformity to simply living, is what this surgery ultimately aims for. Not the number on the X-ray. Not the Cobb angle correction. The person living in the body, fully and without the constant diminishment of a condition that had come to define the edges of their existence.

CHAPTER EIGHTEEN:

LONG-TERM OUTCOMES — WHAT THE EVIDENCE SHOWS

What happens in the years and decades after scoliosis surgery? This is the question that ultimately matters most to patients and families making surgical decisions, and one that decades of rigorous follow-up research have produced increasingly confident answers to. This chapter synthesises that evidence across the domains that matter most: the durability of curve correction, quality of life, pain, pulmonary function, physical activity and sport, pregnancy and reproductive outcomes, and the long-term health of the spine adjacent to the fusion.

DURABILITY OF CURVE CORRECTION — THE TWENTY-YEAR VIEW

The fundamental question about any scoliosis surgery is whether the correction achieved at the time of the procedure persists over the long term. The evidence across multiple well-conducted long-term follow-up studies, some following patients for 20 to 25 years after adolescent idiopathic scoliosis surgery, is reassuring.

Curve correction achieved with modern posterior pedicle screw instrumentation averages approximately 60 to 75 percent of the preoperative Cobb angle. A 60-degree curve is typically corrected to 15 to 24 degrees. Long-term radiographic follow-up demonstrates that this correction is well-maintained, with loss of correction averaging less than five degrees over 10 to 20 year follow-up periods in major published series. This modest loss of correction is clinically inconsequential in the vast majority of patients.

Curves in the unfused segments adjacent to the fusion are monitored over time. In adolescent idiopathic scoliosis, unfused compensatory curves typically improve or stabilise after surgical correction of the primary structural curve, reflecting the restoration of overall spinal balance. Progressive deformity in previously unfused segments is uncommon in the well-planned fusion.

QUALITY OF LIFE — WHAT PATIENTS REPORT

Patient-reported outcomes provide the most clinically relevant picture of surgical benefit. The Scoliosis Research Society's validated outcome questionnaire, used across large cohort studies with long follow-up, demonstrates consistent and significant improvements in all measured domains after successful surgical correction.

The self-image domain shows the largest magnitude of improvement and the most durable benefit in published long-term series. Pain scores improve significantly and remain improved at long-term follow-up. Function scores improve as physical activity is restored and maintained. Mental health scores improve in parallel with physical improvement, reflecting the genuine psychological burden that significant scoliosis imposes and the relief that successful treatment provides.

Comparative studies examining quality of life in surgically treated versus untreated patients with equivalent initial curve magnitudes followed for 20 to 25 years have consistently found superior outcomes in the surgically treated group across most measured domains. The benefit of surgery is most clearly demonstrated in patients who had curves of 50 degrees or greater at skeletal maturity, where the natural history without treatment involves progressive deterioration that surgery effectively prevents.

Patient satisfaction at long-term follow-up after adolescent idiopathic scoliosis surgery is consistently reported at 85 to 95 percent across major published series, with patients reporting that they would make the same decision again. This is among the highest patient satisfaction rates documented for any major elective surgical procedure.

PAIN OUTCOMES OVER DECADES

Back pain is universal in the human population, and patients after scoliosis surgery are not immune to it. The meaningful question is whether their long-term pain burden is better than it would have been without treatment.

The evidence is generally favourable. Long-term follow-up studies of patients after adolescent idiopathic scoliosis surgery report pain scores broadly similar to age-matched general population comparators, and substantially better than comparable untreated patients with similar initial curve magnitudes. The proportion of patients with disabling chronic back pain is significantly lower in surgically treated cohorts than in comparable untreated cohorts followed over the same period.

For adult degenerative scoliosis surgery, pain outcomes are more variable and are critically dependent on the quality of sagittal balance achieved. Studies consistently demonstrate that sagittal balance restoration is the single most powerful predictor of patient-reported pain and functional outcomes after adult spinal deformity surgery. Patients in whom excellent sagittal balance is achieved report dramatically better pain and function outcomes than those in whom balance is suboptimal, even when the coronal correction appears equivalent. This is why sagittal balance is such a central focus of surgical planning and execution in adult deformity surgery.

PULMONARY FUNCTION — BREATHING FOR LIFE

The long-term respiratory consequences of scoliosis and its surgical treatment are particularly important for patients with large thoracic curves. The thoracic cage deformity produced by severe thoracic scoliosis mechanically impairs lung expansion, and in historical series of patients with untreated severe curves, progressive respiratory compromise and shortened life expectancy were documented.

Surgical correction of thoracic scoliosis effectively prevents this progressive pulmonary deterioration. Long-term follow-up studies demonstrate that treated patients maintain pulmonary function over decades at levels substantially better than comparable untreated patients. In some studies, modest improvement in forced vital capacity is documented in the first year or two after surgery.

The respiratory benefit of surgery is greatest when intervention occurs before significant pulmonary compromise has developed. This provides one of the clearest medical arguments for appropriately timed intervention rather than indefinite observation in patients with progressive thoracic scoliosis approaching or exceeding the surgical threshold.

PHYSICAL ACTIVITY, SPORT, AND OCCUPATIONAL OUTCOMES

The evidence on long-term physical activity and occupational function after scoliosis surgery is among the most practically important for patients and families making decisions.

Physical activity participation rates in patients after adolescent idiopathic scoliosis surgery are broadly comparable to age-matched general population comparators at long-term follow-up. Recreational sport participation, competitive sport participation, and high-intensity physical activity are all achievable after well-performed scoliosis fusion. Multiple published studies have demonstrated return to competitive athletics, including elite-level performance, after scoliosis surgery.

Occupational outcomes are similarly favourable. Long-term employment rates, occupational categories, and work-related disability in surgically treated scoliosis patients do not differ significantly from age-matched general population data. Patients after scoliosis surgery work across the full spectrum of occupational demands, including physically demanding manual trades, and achieve occupational success and satisfaction at rates comparable to their peers.

PREGNANCY AND REPRODUCTIVE OUTCOMES

Female patients who underwent scoliosis surgery in adolescence or young adulthood frequently ask about the implications for future pregnancy, and the evidence is reassuring.

Fertility is not adversely affected by scoliosis surgery. Pregnancy rates in women who have had spinal fusion are comparable to those in the general female population. Pregnancy outcomes including rates of normal vaginal delivery and neonatal outcomes are broadly comparable to population norms. Some studies report a modestly higher caesarean rate in women with long fusions involving the lumbar spine, likely reflecting pelvic mobility considerations, but this is not universal and does not indicate a pregnancy complication.

Epidural anaesthesia for labour remains possible after scoliosis fusion in most cases. The technical challenge is greater when the fusion includes lumbar levels, and the expertise of a senior obstetric anaesthetist familiar with managing these cases is important. Women who have had scoliosis surgery should inform their obstetrician at the beginning of pregnancy so that appropriate planning for both obstetric and anaesthetic management can be made.

ADJACENT SEGMENT HEALTH

Adjacent segment disease, meaning degenerative changes in the spinal levels immediately above or below the fused construct, is a recognised long-term consideration following spinal fusion. The immobile fused construct transfers mechanical demand to the adjacent mobile segments, which must compensate for the loss of motion at the fused levels. The clinical significance of adjacent segment changes varies considerably. Many patients show radiographic evidence of adjacent segment degeneration at long-term follow-up without experiencing any related symptoms. Symptomatic adjacent segment disease requiring additional surgical intervention occurs in an estimated 5 to 15 percent of patients over a 10 to 20-year follow-up period.

Risk of adjacent segment disease is higher in adult patients whose adjacent segments show pre-existing degenerative changes at the time of primary surgery, in patients with suboptimal sagittal balance, and when the ends of the fusion are positioned at biomechanically disadvantaged levels. Minimising fusion length by including only the vertebrae necessary to achieve stable correction, and achieving excellent overall spinal balance, are the primary surgical strategies for reducing adjacent segment disease risk.

FROM THE SURGEON'S DESK

The most meaningful conversations I have with patients are not in the pre-operative consultation room, important as those conversations are. They are at the five-year and ten-year follow-up appointments.

I sit across from someone who came to me perhaps decades ago, uncertain and frightened, and I see them as a person who has simply lived their life. Working, travelling, parenting, pursuing the activities they love. The surgery has become simply something that happened, not the defining feature of their life that it felt like at the time.

The evidence I have presented in this chapter supports what I see. Scoliosis surgery, performed well for the right patient at the right time, produces corrections that last, quality of life improvements that are sustained, and functional outcomes that enable full participation in life. That is not a guarantee. Medicine never guarantees outcomes. But it is a well-founded expectation, built on decades of rigorously collected data from tens of thousands of patients followed for decades.

I would not have dedicated my career to this work if I did not believe in it. And the evidence gives me every reason to continue believing.

Part Six

Questions And Answers

Chapter Nineteen:

Frequently Asked Questions

Over many years in surgical practice, certain questions are asked again and again in consultations, follow-up appointments, and pre-operative communications. This chapter collects the most common and gathers direct, honest answers in one accessible place.

Will my implants set off airport security alarms?

Modern titanium spinal implants are not significantly ferromagnetic and do not typically trigger standard electromagnetic walkthrough metal detectors. However, millimetre-wave body scanners increasingly used at international airports may visually detect the implants as a density within the body image. In practice, you may occasionally be asked to step aside for additional screening, most commonly at major international airports with the most advanced scanner systems.

Carrying a medical implant card identifying the nature and location of your spinal instrumentation is recommended. Many airports have designated procedures for passengers with implanted medical devices, and the card provides a clear and credible explanation that resolves any security concern quickly. Most patients with modern titanium implants report that air travel, after an initial period of occasional additional screening, becomes entirely routine.

Can I have MRI scans after surgery?

Yes, and this is an important reassurance. Modern titanium spinal implants are MRI-compatible. They are not ferromagnetic in a clinically meaningful sense, do not move in response to the magnetic fields used in MRI, and do not heat dangerously during scanning. You can safely undergo MRI of any body part after scoliosis surgery.

The practical consideration is image quality rather than safety. Metal implants create artefact, meaning a zone of image distortion, in the MRI image in the immediate vicinity of the metal. This can limit the diagnostic quality of MRI images of the operated spinal segment itself but does not affect imaging of other body regions. Your radiologist will account for this in planning the scan protocol and interpreting the images.

Always inform the MRI team about your spinal implants before any scan. This is routine and important information for scan planning.

How much flexibility will I lose?

Honestly, the loss of flexibility after fusion depends on how many vertebral levels are included and where the fusion sits. Fused segments cannot contribute to spinal range of motion, and overall spinal mobility is reduced proportionally.

The impact on daily function, however, is often significantly less than patients fear before surgery. The thoracic spine contributes relatively little to the functional movements most important in daily life: bending forward to pick things up, and rotation for daily tasks. These movements are primarily generated by the hip joints and the lumbar spine. Patients with thoracic fusions frequently report at long-term follow-up that they are barely aware of any restriction in their normal daily activities.

Lumbar fusions have a more noticeable impact on forward bending and rotation of the lower trunk. Patients with long lumbar fusions will notice a reduced ability to bend at the waist and will adapt certain activities accordingly, most importantly learning to bend by hinging at the hips with a straight back rather than rounding the lumbar spine.

The large majority of patients adapt well to the changes in their functional mobility and report, at long-term follow-up, that the restriction is manageable and far outweighed by the benefits of the surgical correction.

Can I become pregnant after scoliosis surgery?

Yes. Fertility is not adversely affected by scoliosis surgery, and pregnancy rates in women who have had spinal fusion are comparable to the general population. Pregnancy after scoliosis fusion is well-tolerated in the vast majority of cases, with obstetric outcomes broadly comparable to population norms.

The main practical considerations are informing your obstetrician about the previous surgery early in the pregnancy, and ensuring your anaesthetic team is aware of the spinal fusion when planning any anaesthesia for labour or delivery. Epidural anaesthesia for labour can generally be provided after scoliosis fusion, though the technical challenge may be greater when the fusion includes lumbar levels, and the expertise of a senior obstetric anaesthetist is important.

Discuss pregnancy planning with your spinal surgeon if you have specific questions about your individual situation.

What if a rod breaks?

Rod fracture is a recognised late complication that typically occurs years after surgery at a stress concentration point in the rod. It presents as new localised back pain, often at the fracture level, sometimes with a subtle change in back contour, and is confirmed by imaging.

The immediate clinical response to discovering a rod fracture should be measured rather than panicked. A fractured rod in a substantially fused spine does not represent a spinal emergency. The developing bony fusion provides structural support even without the intact rod. The fracture does indicate, however, that fusion has not been completed at the affected level, and without the full rod support, progressive loss of correction may occur there over time.

Management depends on symptoms, the degree of fusion at the fracture level and adjacent levels, and the overall clinical picture. Some fractures in largely fused constructs with minimal symptoms can be observed. Those associated with significant pain, pseudarthrosis at the fracture level, or progressive deformity typically require revision surgery to replace the rod and augment the fusion biology.

Why do I still have some back pain after what appeared to be a successful operation?

Some degree of residual or intermittent back discomfort after major spinal surgery is common and does not indicate that the operation was unsuccessful. The paraspinal muscles, significantly disrupted during surgery, take many months to fully recover and regenerate their pre-operative strength and function. During this extended recovery period, muscular discomfort, stiffness, and aching are normal features.

Biomechanical adaptation also contributes. As the spine adjusts to its new structural configuration and the adjacent unfused segments adapt to their changed mechanical role, discomfort can accompany the adaptive process.

Persistent, worsening, or new pain after surgery, particularly pain that is increasing rather than gradually improving, pain associated with any new neurological symptoms, or pain clearly localised to a specific spinal level, warrants assessment by your surgical team. Imaging can identify specific causes including pseudarthrosis or adjacent segment problems that may benefit from targeted treatment.

How long will the implants last?

Spinal fusion implants do not have a lifespan in the same sense as joint replacement implants such as hip or knee replacements. Hip replacements articulate, meaning the components move against each other and wear over time, requiring revision after 15 to 20 years in many patients. Spinal fusion implants, once the fusion is solid, are supported by bone and do not bear cyclical loads in the same way. Well-fused spinal implants can remain in place indefinitely.

The situations that may require revision of spinal implants are those described in the complications and revision chapters: pseudarthrosis leading to implant fatigue and fracture, junctional failure requiring extension of the construct, or specific implant problems such as a prominent screw causing local discomfort at the wound surface. None of these are related to the inherent lifespan of the titanium implant material itself.

Is it normal to feel tearful and emotional during recovery?

Completely and entirely normal. Emotional responses during recovery including tearfulness, low mood, anxiety, irritability, and frustration are nearly universal after major surgery and reflect a combination of physiological and psychological factors. The inflammatory stress response to surgery, the effects of opioid medications, disrupted sleep, reduced independence and autonomy, and the replacement of purposeful pre-operative focus with the slower pace of recovery all contribute.

These emotions typically improve progressively and naturally as pain decreases, function returns, and recovery milestones accumulate. If emotional difficulty feels severe, is not improving over the first few weeks, or feels like it is worsening rather than getting better, this should be discussed with your surgical or general medical team. Targeted psychological support during recovery is available and effective, and using it is a sign of intelligent self-care.

What is the most important thing I can do for my outcome?

Engage fully and consistently with rehabilitation from the first day through the full twelve months and beyond. The surgery creates the structural correction. What you do with the recovery determines how completely and quickly you build on that correction.

Walk every day, increasing progressively. Do your physiotherapy exercises. Eat well, particularly for protein and bone-supporting nutrients. Do not smoke. Sleep as well as you can. Report any concerning symptoms promptly rather than waiting. Be patient with the biological timeline. And approach the year of recovery with the same commitment you brought to the decision to have surgery in the first place.

The patients who achieve the best long-term outcomes are consistently those who engage most fully with the recovery process and who refuse to let the surgery be the ceiling of what they believe they are capable of.

Part Seven

Additional Resources

CHAPTER TWENTY:

BRACING — UNDERSTANDING THE PATH MANY PATIENTS TRAVEL FIRST

For many patients who eventually undergo scoliosis surgery, bracing was part of their journey before surgery became necessary. For others, bracing was tried and did not prevent progression, and the experience of bracing shapes how they feel about the decision to proceed with surgery. For families of younger children who may face bracing in the future, understanding this treatment in depth provides important context for the overall scoliosis treatment pathway. This chapter is dedicated to explaining bracing thoroughly: what it is, how it works, what the evidence says about its effectiveness, what the experience of wearing a brace involves, and how bracing relates to the eventual decision about surgery.

THE PURPOSE OF BRACING

Bracing is a non-surgical treatment used in growing patients with moderate scoliosis curves, with the specific goal of preventing curve progression during the remaining period of skeletal growth. It is essential to understand from the outset what bracing can and cannot do. Bracing does not correct an existing curve in the sense of making it smaller. What bracing does is apply external corrective forces to the growing spine in a way that, according to the evidence, significantly reduces the probability that the curve will progress to the point where surgery becomes necessary.

This distinction matters enormously for how patients and families understand the bracing experience. A successful course of bracing is one in which the curve at the end of treatment, when growth is complete, is similar to or only modestly larger than the curve at the start of bracing. This is success, even though to a parent looking at X-rays that show "the same number," it can initially feel like nothing has been achieved. In reality, without the brace, the curve would very likely have progressed substantially further, potentially into the surgical range.

THE EVIDENCE FOR BRACING — THE BrAIST STUDY

For many years, the effectiveness of bracing was debated within the medical community, with some clinicians and researchers questioning whether braces achieved anything beyond what would have happened with observation alone. This uncertainty was resolved by a landmark study called BrAIST, the Bracing in Adolescent Idiopathic Scoliosis Trial, published in the New England Journal of Medicine.

The BrAIST study was a randomised controlled trial, the gold standard of medical evidence, that compared bracing to observation in adolescents with moderate idiopathic scoliosis at high risk of progression. The results were striking. In the observation group, approximately 48 percent of patients progressed to the surgical threshold by skeletal maturity. In the bracing group, this fell to approximately 28 percent. Furthermore, the study demonstrated a clear dose-response relationship: patients who wore their braces for more hours per day had progressively lower rates of progression to surgical thresholds. Patients who achieved more than 12.9 hours of wear per day had success rates exceeding 90 to 95 percent.

This study fundamentally changed the conversation about bracing. It provided definitive evidence that bracing works, that its effectiveness is directly related to how consistently it is worn, and that the commitment required from patients and families to achieve high-hours compliance is genuinely worthwhile in terms of avoiding surgery.

TYPES OF BRACES

Several brace designs are used in contemporary practice, each with specific characteristics suited to different curve patterns.

The Boston brace, also known as a thoracolumbosacral orthosis or TLSO, is one of the most widely used designs. It is a custom-moulded plastic brace that extends from below the armpits to the hips, with internal pads positioned to apply corrective pressure to specific points of the curve while creating space on the opposite side for the spine to move into. The Boston brace is moulded from a plaster cast or, increasingly, from a three-dimensional scan of the patient's torso, allowing for precise customisation.

The Rigo-Cheneau brace represents a more recent evolution in brace design, incorporating principles of three-dimensional correction that address not just the lateral curve but also the rotational component of scoliosis. These braces are designed with asymmetric reliefs and pressure points calculated to encourage the spine to derotate as well as straighten, and many specialist centres now favour this type of brace design for its more comprehensive approach to the three-dimensional nature of scoliosis.

The Milwaukee brace, historically significant as one of the earliest effective scoliosis braces, includes a neck ring and extends higher on the torso than the Boston brace. It is now used less frequently than TLSO designs but remains appropriate for curves with a significant component in the upper thoracic spine that TLSO braces cannot adequately address.

Nighttime bracing, including designs such as the Providence brace, applies more aggressive overcorrection forces that can only be tolerated while lying down, worn exclusively during sleep. These braces may be appropriate for smaller curves with specific characteristics, offering the advantage of not affecting the patient's daytime appearance or activities, though the evidence base for nighttime bracing alone in larger curves is less robust than for full-time TLSO bracing.

THE BRACE FITTING PROCESS

The process of obtaining a brace begins with a detailed assessment of the curve, including its location, magnitude, flexibility, and the specific anatomical features that will guide brace design. Many centres now use surface scanning technology to capture a three-dimensional image of the patient's torso, which is used to design the brace digitally before manufacture, replacing the traditional plaster casting process in many settings.

Once manufactured, the brace undergoes a fitting process during which an orthotist, a specialist in orthopaedic devices, adjusts the brace to ensure appropriate fit, comfort, and the application of corrective forces at the intended locations. This fitting process often requires several iterations, and it is normal for adjustments to be needed in the early weeks of wear as the patient and the orthotist refine the fit.

An in-brace X-ray, taken with the patient wearing the brace, is typically obtained to confirm that the brace is achieving the intended correction. A well-fitted brace should produce a measurable reduction in the Cobb angle compared to the out-of-brace measurement, demonstrating that the corrective forces are being applied effectively.

THE EXPERIENCE OF WEARING A BRACE

For patients, particularly adolescents, the experience of wearing a brace for 16 to 23 hours per day is significant and deserves honest discussion. The brace is a rigid plastic shell that must be worn under clothing, which can affect how clothes fit and can be warm, particularly in hot climates or seasons. Adjustment to wearing the brace typically takes several weeks, during which patients commonly experience some skin irritation at pressure points, difficulty finding comfortable positions for sitting and sleeping, and the social adjustment of having a visible difference under clothing.

Most centres recommend a gradual increase in wearing time over the first one to two weeks, allowing the skin and the patient to adjust progressively rather than attempting full-time wear immediately. Skin care is important, including keeping the skin clean and dry, wearing a thin, seamless cotton garment under the brace to reduce friction, and monitoring for any areas of persistent redness or skin breakdown that may indicate the brace needs adjustment.

Despite these challenges, the evidence is clear that most adolescents adapt successfully to brace wear, particularly when they understand why it matters and when they receive support from family, school, and healthcare providers in navigating the practical and social aspects of the experience.

WHEN BRACING DOES NOT PREVENT PROGRESSION

For some patients, despite good compliance with bracing, the curve progresses to the surgical threshold regardless. This outcome can be emotionally difficult for patients and families who have invested significant effort in the bracing programme, and it is important to address this directly.

Progression despite good bracing compliance is not a failure of the patient or family. It reflects the underlying biological reality that, in some patients, the forces driving curve progression are stronger than what bracing, even optimally applied, can resist. The BrAIST study itself demonstrated that even with excellent compliance, a minority of patients progressed despite bracing. This is a recognised feature of the natural history of scoliosis in a subset of patients, not evidence of inadequate effort.

For patients in this situation, the transition from bracing to surgical consideration can carry a particular emotional weight, sometimes including a sense that the years of bracing were wasted. This is not an accurate way to understand the situation. The bracing period, even when it did not ultimately prevent the need for surgery, may have delayed progression, allowing the patient to reach a stage of greater skeletal maturity before surgery, which can affect surgical planning and timing in beneficial ways. The bracing period was not wasted; it was part of a carefully managed treatment pathway that, for this particular patient, ultimately required the additional step of surgical correction.

FROM THE SURGEON'S DESK

I see many patients who arrive at the surgical consultation having spent years in a brace, and I want to address something directly to them and their families: the years of bracing were not a failure, and they were not wasted.

Bracing is the appropriate evidence-based treatment for moderate progressive curves in growing patients, and the decision to brace was the right decision at the time it was made, based on the information available then. If the curve has now progressed to a point where surgery is recommended, that does not retrospectively make the bracing decision wrong. It means that for this particular patient, with this particular biology, the curve was always going to require surgical correction eventually, and bracing may have delayed that point, allowing growth and maturity to progress in ways that can be beneficial for surgical planning.

I have huge respect for the families who navigate years of brace wear with their children. It requires patience, persistence, and often difficult conversations about a visible difference during years when fitting in matters enormously to young people. That effort was not wasted. It was part of the careful, evidence-based management of a condition that, for some patients, ultimately benefits from surgical correction as the next and final step.

CHAPTER TWENTY-ONE:

A GUIDE FOR CAREGIVERS AND FAMILY MEMBERS

While the focus of this book has rightly been on the patient undergoing scoliosis surgery, the experience of surgery extends well beyond the individual patient to encompass parents, partners, siblings, and the wider circle of family and friends who provide support throughout the journey. This chapter is written specifically for those caregivers: the people who will be driving to appointments, managing schedules, providing physical care during recovery, and carrying their own emotional load throughout the process.

THE CAREGIVER'S EMOTIONAL EXPERIENCE

Caring for someone undergoing major surgery is itself an emotionally significant experience, and caregivers frequently report that their own emotional needs are overlooked in a system that, understandably, focuses its attention on the patient.

For parents of children and adolescents undergoing scoliosis surgery, the emotional experience often spans years before the surgical decision is even reached. Parents who have been managing a child's scoliosis through the diagnostic process, the monitoring appointments, potentially the bracing years, and now the surgical decision, carry an accumulated emotional weight that deserves acknowledgment. The anxiety of watching your child face a major operation, the responsibility of having made or supported treatment decisions on their behalf, and the practical burden of coordinating care all contribute to a significant caregiver experience.

For partners and spouses of adult patients, the experience involves navigating a partner's major surgery and recovery while often also managing household responsibilities, potentially childcare, and their own work commitments, all while providing emotional and physical support during the recovery period.

For siblings, particularly younger siblings of paediatric patients, the experience can include disruption to normal family routines, anxiety about a sibling undergoing surgery, and sometimes feelings of being overlooked during a period when parental attention is necessarily focused on the patient.

Recognising and validating these experiences is important. Caregivers who acknowledge their own emotional responses, who seek support when needed, and who attend to their own wellbeing are better able to sustain the support they provide over what can be a demanding period.

PRACTICAL PREPARATION FOR CAREGIVERS

The practical role of caregivers spans the entire surgical journey, and thoughtful preparation makes this role considerably more manageable.

In the pre-operative period, caregivers often take on the role of information gatherer and organiser, attending appointments, taking notes, helping to formulate questions, and helping the patient process and remember information provided by the medical team. Having a shared system for tracking appointments, questions, and information, whether a notebook, a shared digital document, or another method that works for your family, reduces the cognitive load on everyone involved.

Practical preparation of the home, as described in Chapter Six, is often primarily the responsibility of caregivers. This includes arranging the sleeping environment, bathroom modifications, and organising the practical support network for the post-operative period.

On the day of surgery itself, caregivers face their own significant emotional experience: the wait during the operation, which for scoliosis surgery can be four to eight hours or more. Having a plan for how to spend this waiting time, whether that means staying at the hospital, going for a walk, or having a support person of your own present, can make this difficult period more manageable. Most hospitals provide updates during long procedures, and knowing what update process to expect can reduce anxiety during the wait.

During the hospital stay, caregivers play an important role in supporting the patient through what can be a difficult few days, while also managing their own need for rest and self-care. It is not necessary, and is often not advisable, for a caregiver to remain at the hospital around the clock. Rested caregivers provide better support than exhausted ones.

SUPPORTING RECOVERY AT HOME

The home recovery period places the most sustained practical demands on caregivers, typically over the first two to six weeks, with a tapering level of support needed over the following months.

Practical care tasks in the early weeks may include assistance with personal care, particularly tasks that involve bending or reaching that the patient cannot yet safely perform, meal preparation, household management, transport to follow-up appointments and physiotherapy, medication management, including ensuring medications are taken on schedule, and general supervision, particularly important in the first days at home when the effects of medications and the early stages of mobility can create fall risks.

Emotional support during this period is equally important. The post-surgical emotional dip described in earlier chapters affects not only patients but can be observed and responded to by attentive caregivers. Simply being present, listening without trying to fix or minimise difficult feelings, and gently encouraging engagement with the recovery programme without being perceived as nagging, are valuable forms of support that caregivers are well-placed to provide.

Encouraging appropriate independence is a balance that caregivers often navigate without explicit guidance. While significant support is needed in the early weeks, recovery also involves a progressive return of independence, and caregivers who recognise and support this progression, rather than inadvertently fostering excessive dependence through over-helping, support the patient's recovery in both functional and psychological terms. The physiotherapy and surgical team can provide guidance on what level of independence is appropriate at each stage, and caregivers are encouraged to ask directly about this.

SUPPORTING ADOLESCENT PATIENTS SPECIFICALLY

Parents of adolescent patients face particular considerations. Adolescence is developmentally a period of increasing independence, and major surgery that necessitates a temporary return to greater dependence on parents can create tension, even when both parties understand it is necessary and temporary.

Respecting the adolescent's developing autonomy within the constraints of the recovery period, involving them in decisions about their own care where appropriate, and communicating openly about the temporary nature of increased dependence can help navigate this tension.

School liaison is an important practical task for parents of school-aged patients. Establishing communication with the school before surgery, providing information about the expected recovery timeline and any necessary accommodations, and maintaining this communication throughout the recovery period helps ensure a smooth return to the educational environment.

Sibling considerations deserve attention. Younger siblings may benefit from age-appropriate explanations of what is happening, reassurance about their own routines and care during the period of focused attention on the patient, and opportunities to be involved in supportive ways that help them feel part of the process rather than excluded from it.

SUPPORTING ADULT PATIENTS

For caregivers of adult patients, the dynamics differ but the support need is equally real. Adult patients facing major surgery often have their own established roles within the family, whether as primary earners, primary caregivers for children or elderly relatives, or in other significant capacities, and the temporary disruption of these roles during recovery can create both practical and emotional challenges.

Open communication about how household responsibilities will be managed during the recovery period, realistic planning for the practical gaps that will need to be filled, and recognition that the recovery timeline, while temporary, genuinely does require months rather than weeks for full functional recovery, all support a smoother adjustment for the whole family unit.

CAREGIVER SELF-CARE

It cannot be emphasised enough that caregivers who attend to their own physical and emotional wellbeing are better able to sustain the support they provide. This is not a luxury or a distraction from the caregiving role; it is a component of it.

Practical self-care includes ensuring adequate sleep, even when this means arranging for others to share overnight responsibilities during the most demanding early period. Maintaining your own routines where possible, including exercise, social connection, and activities that support your own wellbeing. Accepting help when it is offered, whether from extended family, friends, or community resources, rather than attempting to manage everything independently. And recognising your own emotional responses to the experience, including anxiety, fatigue, and sometimes resentment or frustration, as normal and worthy of attention rather than feelings to be suppressed.

If you find that your own wellbeing is significantly affected, whether through persistent anxiety, exhaustion, or low mood, seeking support for yourself, whether through your own healthcare provider, counselling services, or caregiver support groups, is appropriate and valuable. Many hospitals and patient organisations offer resources specifically for caregivers and family members navigating major surgery.

FROM THE SURGEON'S DESK

I have learned over the years to pay attention to the caregivers in the room, not just the patient. The parent who has driven for two hours to bring their child to this appointment. The spouse who has rearranged their work schedule around hospital visits. The adult child who is supporting an elderly parent through a major operation.

These people carry a significant burden, and they often feel that their role is to be strong and supportive for the patient, without space for their own concerns. I try, in my consultations, to acknowledge directly what I see: that this is hard for you too, that your role matters, and that taking care of yourself is part of taking care of your loved one.

Recovery from major surgery is, in the truest sense, a family experience. The patient is at its centre, but the family around them carries much of the practical and emotional weight that makes recovery possible. That contribution deserves to be seen and valued, and I hope this chapter has done some justice to it.

CHAPTER TWENTY-TWO:

UNDERSTANDING YOUR IMAGING REPORTS

Throughout the scoliosis journey, imaging reports are among the documents you will encounter most frequently, and they are often written in dense medical terminology that can feel impenetrable to patients and families. This chapter is designed to help you read and understand your own imaging reports, so that the information that is, after all, about your own body becomes accessible to you rather than remaining a collection of unfamiliar terms.

THE STRUCTURE OF A TYPICAL X-RAY REPORT

A standard radiology report for a scoliosis X-ray typically follows a consistent structure: a clinical history section summarising why the imaging was requested, a technique section describing what views were obtained, a findings section describing what is seen on the images, and an impression or conclusion section summarising the key points.

The findings section is usually the most detailed and the most likely to contain unfamiliar terminology. For a scoliosis X-ray, you can expect to see references to the Cobb angle measurements for each significant curve, described by the levels involved, for example "a right thoracic curve from T5 to T12 measuring 52 degrees." You may see references to coronal balance, describing whether the trunk is centred over the pelvis or shifted to one side. You may see references to sagittal alignment, describing the thoracic kyphosis and lumbar lordosis measurements. In growing patients, the Risser sign will typically be reported, providing the skeletal maturity grading from 0 to 5.

UNDERSTANDING CURVE DESCRIPTIONS

Curves are typically described by their location, their direction, and their magnitude. The location is given by the vertebral levels at the top and bottom of the curve, for example T5 to T12 indicates a curve extending from the fifth thoracic vertebra to the twelfth thoracic vertebra. The direction is described as either right or left, referring to the direction of the convexity, meaning the outward-bulging side of the curve. A right thoracic curve, for instance, bulges toward the patient's right side. The magnitude is the Cobb angle in degrees, as discussed extensively in earlier chapters.

When multiple curves are present, they are typically listed in order, often with a description of the overall pattern, such as "double major curve pattern" indicating two roughly equal structural curves, often one thoracic and one lumbar, curving in opposite directions.

UNDERSTANDING MRI REPORTS

MRI reports for the spine contain additional terminology relating to the soft tissue structures visible on this type of imaging. You may encounter references to disc levels, described using the convention of the two adjacent vertebrae, for example "L4-L5" referring to the disc between the fourth and fifth lumbar vertebrae. Descriptions of discs may include terms such as desiccated, referring to loss of the normal water content and signal intensity of the disc, indicating degeneration, and bulge or herniation, referring to displacement of disc material beyond its normal boundaries.

References to the spinal cord may include descriptions of its position, its signal characteristics, and specifically in the context of scoliosis evaluation, whether any abnormalities such as a syrinx, a fluid-filled cavity within the cord, are identified.

References to the nerve roots and foramina may describe whether these structures appear compressed or narrowed, using terms such as foraminal stenosis to describe narrowing of the nerve root exit channels.

UNDERSTANDING CT REPORTS

CT reports focus on the bony anatomy in greater detail than X-ray or MRI. In the context of scoliosis, CT reports may describe the precise anatomy of vertebrae in cases of congenital scoliosis, the position and integrity of any existing surgical implants in revision cases, and detailed measurements of bone density in some protocols.

WHAT TO ASK YOUR SURGEON ABOUT YOUR IMAGING

Rather than attempting to fully interpret imaging reports independently, the most valuable approach is to use your understanding of the terminology to ask informed questions of your surgical team. Useful questions include asking your surgeon to show you on the actual images, not just describe verbally, where your curve is and how it has changed over time if previous imaging is available. Asking what the specific numbers mean for your situation, since the same Cobb angle can have different implications depending on other factors discussed throughout this book. And asking whether any findings on MRI or CT, if performed, have specific implications for your surgical planning.

FROM THE SURGEON'S DESK

I always try to show patients their own images rather than simply reading them a report. There is something powerful about seeing your own spine, understanding where the curve begins and ends, seeing the rotation that the report describes in technical language. It transforms abstract numbers into a concrete understanding of your own anatomy.

If your surgical team has not shown you your own images, ask them to. It is your body, and seeing it is one of the most valuable parts of becoming truly informed about your own care.

CHAPTER TWENTY-THREE:

A PRACTICAL NUTRITION GUIDE FOR SURGERY AND RECOVERY

Chapter Seven introduced the principles of nutrition in the pre-operative period. This chapter provides practical, applied guidance for both the pre-operative weeks and the post-operative recovery period, including sample meal structures designed to meet the elevated protein and micronutrient requirements that surgical healing demands.

DAILY PROTEIN TARGETS IN PRACTICE

Recall that the target protein intake for surgical patients is approximately 1.2 to 1.5 grams per kilogram of body weight per day. For practical purposes, this means most adult patients should aim for somewhere between 80 and 120 grams of protein daily, distributed across three to five eating occasions.

A practical way to think about this is in terms of protein "units" at each meal. A palm-sized portion of meat, fish, or poultry provides approximately 25 to 30 grams of protein. Two large eggs provide approximately 12 to 14 grams. A cup of Greek yoghurt provides approximately 15 to 20 grams. A cup of cooked lentils or beans provides approximately 15 to 18 grams. A standard scoop of protein powder provides approximately 20 to 25 grams. Aiming for two to three of these protein units at each main meal, plus one at a snack, comfortably achieves the daily target for most patients.

SAMPLE DAILY MEAL STRUCTURE — PRE-OPERATIVE

Breakfast might include scrambled eggs with whole grain toast and a side of fruit, or Greek yoghurt with berries and a sprinkle of nuts and seeds, providing both protein and the vitamin C that supports collagen formation and iron absorption.

A mid-morning snack might include a handful of nuts with a piece of fruit, or a protein smoothie made with milk or a fortified plant milk, a scoop of protein powder, and frozen fruit.

Lunch might centre on a portion of grilled chicken, fish, or a plant-based protein such as tofu or tempeh, served with a substantial portion of vegetables and a wholegrain such as brown rice or quinoa.

An afternoon snack could be cottage cheese with fruit, or hummus with vegetable sticks and wholegrain crackers.

Dinner might include a lean meat, fish, or legume-based main course, again with a generous portion of vegetables and a wholegrain or starchy vegetable such as sweet potato.

An evening snack, particularly important for patients who struggle to meet protein targets during the day, might include a small portion of cheese, a glass of milk, or a small protein shake.

SAMPLE MEAL STRUCTURE — EARLY POST-OPERATIVE PERIOD

In the first few days after surgery, appetite is often reduced, and the focus should be on small, frequent, nutrient-dense intake rather than large meals. Smoothies and shakes are particularly valuable in this period because they allow significant nutritional intake, including protein, fruit, and even vegetables, in a form that is easy to consume when appetite is limited.

A recovery smoothie might combine milk or fortified plant milk, a scoop of protein powder, a banana for easy-to-digest carbohydrate and potassium, a handful of spinach for iron and folate, blended until smooth. This single drink can provide 25 to 30 grams of protein along with meaningful micronutrient content, in a form that requires minimal effort to consume.

Soups, particularly those made with a base of bone broth or with added protein from lentils, beans, or shredded meat, are warming, easy to digest, and can be nutrient-dense. Soft, easily chewed proteins such as scrambled eggs, fish, slow-cooked meat, yoghurt, and well-cooked legumes are appropriate when appetite begins to return but the energy for substantial chewing or large meals is still limited.

ADDRESSING CONSTIPATION THROUGH DIET

As discussed in earlier chapters, constipation related to opioid medications is a near-universal feature of the early recovery period, and dietary measures complement the stool softeners and laxatives that will be prescribed.

Fluid intake should be generous, aiming for at least two litres of fluid daily unless otherwise advised, as adequate hydration is essential for normal bowel function. Fibre-rich foods including whole fruits with skins where appropriate, vegetables, whole grains, and legumes support bowel regularity, though very high-fibre intake without adequate fluid can worsen rather than improve constipation, so the two should be increased together. Prunes and prune juice have a long-recognised mild laxative effect and are a useful addition to the daily diet during the early recovery period.

SUPPLEMENTS WORTH DISCUSSING WITH YOUR TEAM

Several supplements are commonly recommended in the perioperative period, though the specific recommendations should always be individualised based on your blood tests and your surgical team's guidance. Vitamin D, often at doses of 1000 to 4000 IU daily, particularly if pre-operative testing identifies deficiency. Calcium, typically aiming for a total dietary and supplemental intake of 1000 to 1200 milligrams daily. Iron, if pre-operative anaemia or low iron stores are identified, in a form and dose determined by your medical team. Vitamin C, which supports collagen synthesis and enhances iron absorption. And a general multivitamin as a safety net for micronutrient adequacy during a period when dietary intake may be irregular.

Always discuss any supplement use with your surgical team, as some supplements, particularly those affecting blood clotting such as fish oil and vitamin E at high doses, need to be stopped before surgery as discussed in Chapter Six.

FROM THE SURGEON'S DESK

Nutrition is one of the few aspects of surgical preparation and recovery that is entirely within the patient's own control, and I have come to believe it deserves far more attention than it traditionally receives in surgical care pathways.

I do not expect patients to become nutrition experts. What I ask is that they take the basic principles seriously: adequate protein, adequate vitamin D and calcium, adequate iron, good hydration, and a generally whole-food-based diet in the weeks before and the months after surgery. These are not difficult or expensive changes for most people, and the evidence that they support better healing is compelling.

CHAPTER TWENTY-FOUR:

CHECKLISTS AND QUESTION GUIDES FOR EVERY STAGE

This chapter consolidates practical checklists and question guides referenced throughout the book into one place for easy reference. Photocopy these pages, write directly in the book, or use them as templates for your own notes.

QUESTIONS FOR YOUR INITIAL SURGICAL CONSULTATION

What is my specific diagnosis, including the type of scoliosis, the Cobb angle of each significant curve, and my skeletal maturity status if relevant. What is the natural history of my specific curve if left untreated, based on the available evidence. What are the treatment options available to me, including observation, bracing if relevant, and surgery, and what is the rationale for the specific recommendation being made. If surgery is recommended, what is the proposed surgical approach and which vertebral levels would be included in the fusion. What degree of correction is realistically anticipated. What are the specific risks relevant to my situation, and how are these risks managed at this institution. How many procedures similar to mine does this surgeon and this institution perform annually. What does the recovery timeline look like, including hospital stay, return to school or work, and return to sport or other activities important to me. What support is available, including physiotherapy, psychological support, and patient education resources. Can I see my own imaging and have it explained to me directly.

QUESTIONS FOR A SECOND OPINION CONSULTATION

Does the second surgeon agree with the diagnosis and the surgical indication. Does the second surgeon agree with the proposed surgical approach and levels, or would they recommend something different, and if so, why. Are there any additional considerations or options that were not discussed in the first consultation. How does the second surgeon's experience and case volume compare for procedures similar to mine.

PRE-OPERATIVE PREPARATION CHECKLIST

Medical: pre-operative blood tests completed, ECG completed if required, anaesthetic consultation attended, any required additional imaging completed, medication review completed with clear instructions about what to stop and when, any necessary vaccinations or other medical preparations addressed, smoking cessation support accessed if relevant, nutritional assessment and any necessary supplementation begun.

Practical: home modifications completed including sleeping arrangement, bathroom adaptations, comfortable seating, support network confirmed for the post-operative weeks, work or school informed and accommodations discussed, prescriptions for post-operative medications arranged in advance where possible, transport arranged for the day of surgery and for discharge, hospital bag packed with essentials.

Psychological: educational materials reviewed including this book, any specific fears or concerns discussed with the surgical team, mindfulness or relaxation techniques practised if planning to use these, support network informed and available for the recovery period.

DAY OF SURGERY CHECKLIST

Fasting instructions followed precisely. Required pre-operative shower completed if instructed. Jewellery, valuables, and nail varnish removed. Comfortable clothing for after surgery packed. Identification and relevant documentation brought. All questions addressed before going to theatre. Support person's contact details confirmed with the hospital for updates during surgery.

DISCHARGE READINESS CHECKLIST

Pain adequately controlled with oral medications. Able to mobilise safely with appropriate aids if needed. Wound care instructions understood. Medication regimen understood, including what to take, when, and for how long. Warning signs to watch for clearly understood. Follow-up appointments scheduled. Home support confirmed and available. Emergency contact information for the surgical team available.

WARNING SIGNS REQUIRING URGENT CONTACT WITH YOUR SURGICAL TEAM

Worsening pain not controlled by prescribed medications. New or worsening weakness, numbness, or tingling in the legs. Any change in bladder or bowel control. Signs of wound infection: increasing redness, warmth, swelling, or discharge, particularly with fever. Fever above 38 degrees Celsius. Significant swelling, redness, or warmth in one or both calves. Chest pain or shortness of breath, which requires emergency assessment.

RECOVERY MILESTONE TRACKER

Use this as a framework for tracking your own progress, recognising that individual timelines vary and these are general guides rather than fixed targets. Day one: first mobilisation with physiotherapy support. Day two to three: drains and catheter removed if applicable, increasing mobility. Day three to seven: discharge from hospital. Week one to two: walking around the house and short distances outside, suture or staple removal. Week two to four: walking 10 to 15 minutes continuously, return to light activities at home. Week four to six: walking 20 to 30 minutes, possible return to driving and sedentary work or school with clearance. Week six to twelve: progression of physiotherapy, possible introduction of swimming and stationary cycling with clearance. Month three to six: expanding activity levels, possible return to non-contact sport with clearance. Month six to twelve: progression toward full activity including contact sport with explicit clearance. Month twelve and beyond: continued long-term follow-up, established active lifestyle.

FROM THE SURGEON'S DESK

I have found that patients who arrive at appointments with written questions, who have thought through their own checklist of practical preparations, and who track their own recovery milestones tend to have a fundamentally different relationship with their care than those who arrive without this preparation.

This is not about being a difficult or demanding patient. It is about being an engaged one. The checklists in this chapter are tools, not requirements, but I have seen consistently that patients who use tools like these feel more in control of a process that can otherwise feel like something happening to them rather than something they are actively participating in.

CHAPTER TWENTY-FIVE:

LIVING WITH SCOLIOSIS BEFORE SURGERY MANAGING DAILY LIFE

For many patients, the period between diagnosis and surgery, sometimes spanning months, sometimes years, is a significant portion of life lived with an untreated or progressing curve. This chapter addresses the practical realities of living with scoliosis during this period: managing symptoms, navigating daily activities, and understanding when changes in your condition should prompt earlier review.

MANAGING DAY-TO-DAY DISCOMFORT

While scoliosis itself does not always cause pain, particularly in adolescents with idiopathic curves, many patients experience some degree of discomfort related to muscular fatigue from the asymmetric postural demands the curve places on the paraspinal muscles. Understanding the source of this discomfort and how to manage it appropriately, without masking signals that should prompt medical review, is useful.

Postural awareness, without becoming preoccupied or anxious about posture, can help reduce muscular fatigue. Simple measures such as taking regular breaks from prolonged sitting, particularly at school desks or workstations, using supportive seating where possible, and avoiding carrying heavy bags on one shoulder for extended periods, can reduce the cumulative muscular strain that contributes to discomfort.

Gentle, regular physical activity, as tolerated and as advised by your treating team, supports muscular health and can reduce discomfort. This is distinct from intensive exercise programmes and should be discussed with your medical team, particularly if you are in a bracing programme with specific activity guidance.

Heat application to fatigued muscles, through a warm bath, heating pad, or similar, can provide symptomatic relief for muscular discomfort related to postural strain. This is a reasonable self-care measure for muscular aching that is consistent with what you have experienced before and does not represent a new or escalating symptom.

WHEN TO SEEK EARLIER REVIEW

While scheduled monitoring appointments are the primary mechanism for tracking your curve over time, certain changes warrant contacting your medical team before your next scheduled appointment. These include a noticeable increase in visible asymmetry, such as a parent or patient noticing that the rib hump, shoulder height difference, or waist asymmetry has become more pronounced since it was last assessed. New or worsening back pain, particularly pain that is persistent, that wakes you at night, or that is associated with any other new symptoms. Any new neurological symptoms including numbness, tingling, weakness, or changes in bladder or bowel function, which, as discussed throughout this book, warrant urgent assessment regardless of the stage of your scoliosis journey. And for growing patients, a noticeable acceleration in height growth, since periods of rapid growth are associated with higher rates of curve progression and may warrant closer monitoring during that period.

NAVIGATING SCHOOL AND SOCIAL LIFE WITH SCOLIOSIS

For adolescent patients, navigating school and social environments while managing scoliosis, and potentially while wearing a brace, presents practical and social challenges that are worth addressing directly.

Physical education and sport participation should be discussed with your medical team, as the appropriate level of participation depends on your specific curve, whether you are bracing, and your individual circumstances. Many patients with scoliosis, including those in bracing programmes, can participate in most physical education activities, sometimes with brace removal for the activity itself if this has been specifically discussed and approved.

Disclosure to peers about scoliosis or brace wear is a personal decision, and there is no single right approach. Some adolescents find that openly discussing their situation with close friends reduces the anxiety of concealment and can result in supportive responses. Others prefer to manage their situation more privately. Both approaches are valid, and the right choice depends on the individual's personality, social context, and comfort level. What is most important is that the adolescent feels they have agency in this decision, rather than it being made for them.

School staff awareness, at least among relevant teachers and school nurses, is generally beneficial, ensuring that any necessary accommodations, such as permission to stand and move during long lessons for brace-wearing students, or awareness of upcoming medical appointments, can be supported without the student needing to explain their situation repeatedly.

THE TRANSITION TO SURGICAL DECISION-MAKING

For patients who have been living with scoliosis for an extended period before surgery becomes the recommendation, the transition to active surgical decision-making can feel like a significant shift, sometimes after years of a more passive monitoring or bracing-focused relationship with the condition.

This transition often brings a mix of emotions: relief that active treatment addressing the underlying problem is now being offered, alongside the anxiety that comes with facing a major operation. Both responses are normal, and the information in this book is intended to support you through exactly this transition, providing the knowledge needed to engage actively with the decisions ahead.

FROM THE SURGEON'S DESK

I see many patients who have lived with their scoliosis for years before our first meeting, and they often arrive with a complex relationship with their condition. For some, scoliosis has become simply a part of their life, something they have adapted to and barely think about day to day, until imaging shows it has progressed to a point requiring active discussion. For others, the years of monitoring have been marked by ongoing anxiety, waiting for the next X-ray, wondering what it will show.

Whatever your relationship with your scoliosis has been up to this point, the consultation where surgery becomes part of the conversation is a meaningful moment, and I try to honour that. It is the point where the years of watching and waiting transition into active decision-making, and that transition deserves the time and care this book and your surgical team aim to provide.

Chapter Twenty-Six:

A Deeper Look At Anaesthesia For Spinal Surgery

Chapter Eleven introduced the experience of anaesthesia for scoliosis surgery from the patient's perspective. This chapter goes deeper into the science and practice of anaesthesia for major spinal surgery, addressing the specific considerations that make spinal deformity anaesthesia a specialised area of practice, and answering some of the more detailed questions patients often have about this aspect of their care.

WHY SPINAL DEFORMITY ANAESTHESIA IS SPECIALISED

Anaesthesia for scoliosis surgery presents a combination of challenges that together justify the involvement of anaesthetists with specific experience in this field, often called neuroanaesthetists or spinal deformity anaesthetists at specialist centres.

The prone position itself, in which the patient lies face-down for the duration of surgery, creates specific physiological considerations. Venous return to the heart, lung mechanics, and the distribution of blood flow are all affected by this position differently than in the more commonly encountered supine position. Anaesthetists experienced in spinal deformity surgery understand these effects deeply and manage the anaesthetic accordingly.

The requirement for intraoperative neurophysiological monitoring places specific constraints on anaesthetic technique. Many anaesthetic agents, particularly inhaled anaesthetic gases at higher concentrations and certain muscle relaxant drugs, can interfere with the signals used for SSEP and MEP monitoring. Anaesthetists managing scoliosis surgery use anaesthetic techniques and drug combinations specifically chosen to maintain adequate anaesthesia and analgesia while preserving the ability to obtain reliable neuromonitoring signals throughout the procedure. This often involves a technique called total intravenous anaesthesia, using intravenous infusions of anaesthetic agents rather than inhaled gases, which has less impact on monitoring signals.

The management of significant blood loss, as discussed in earlier chapters, requires anaesthetic expertise in blood conservation techniques, fluid management, and transfusion decision-making throughout what can be a lengthy procedure.

Controlled hypotension, deliberately maintaining blood pressure at the lower end of the normal range during specific phases of surgery to reduce blood loss, requires careful balancing against the need to maintain adequate blood flow to the spinal cord, particularly during the phases of surgery when correction forces are being applied and the spinal cord may already be under some degree of mechanical stress.

Temperature management during long procedures is another specific consideration. Maintaining normal body temperature, called normothermia, throughout a procedure that may last many hours requires active warming measures, as patients lose heat readily during long surgical procedures, and hypothermia adversely affects clotting, immune function, and drug metabolism.

THE PRE-OPERATIVE ANAESTHETIC ASSESSMENT IN DETAIL

The pre-operative anaesthetic consultation, introduced in Chapter Six, deserves further explanation of what is being assessed and why.

Airway assessment evaluates how easily the anaesthetist anticipates being able to manage your airway during anaesthesia, including placing the breathing tube. Most patients have airways that present no particular difficulty, but specific anatomical features are assessed and any anticipated difficulty is planned for in advance.

Cardiovascular assessment evaluates your heart's ability to tolerate the physiological demands of major surgery, including the blood loss and fluid shifts involved. For most adolescent and young adult patients, this assessment confirms normal cardiovascular function.

For older adult patients, particularly those with any cardiac history, this assessment may be more detailed and may involve additional tests such as echocardiography.

Respiratory assessment is particularly relevant for patients with significant thoracic curves, where lung function may already be affected by the chest wall deformity. Pulmonary function testing, if performed, informs the anaesthetic plan, particularly regarding post-operative respiratory management.

Risk stratification tools, such as the American Society of Anesthesiologists physical status classification, provide a standardised framework for communicating a patient's overall fitness for anaesthesia among the surgical team, though this single classification does not capture every relevant detail of an individual's situation and is one input among many into the overall anaesthetic plan.

UNDERSTANDING THE DRUGS USED

While the specific anaesthetic protocol varies between institutions and individual patients, understanding the broad categories of drugs used can help demystify the process.

Induction agents, given intravenously to rapidly produce unconsciousness at the start of anaesthesia, work within seconds by affecting specific receptors in the brain that govern consciousness.

Maintenance agents keep the patient unconscious throughout the procedure, either through continued intravenous infusion, total intravenous anaesthesia, or through inhaled anaesthetic gases, with the choice influenced by the need to preserve neuromonitoring signal quality as discussed above.

Analgesic agents, including opioids given intraoperatively, manage the pain response to surgery and contribute to post-operative pain control when their effects continue into the early recovery period.

Muscle relaxant agents may be used at specific points, particularly to facilitate placement of the breathing tube at the start of anaesthesia, but their use during the procedure itself is carefully managed because complete muscle relaxation can interfere with motor evoked potential monitoring, which requires the ability to detect muscle responses to stimulation.

Tranexamic acid, discussed in the context of blood conservation, is administered as part of the anaesthetic protocol to reduce blood loss throughout the procedure.

WAKING UP AND THE IMMEDIATE POST-ANAESTHETIC PERIOD

The process of emergence from anaesthesia, transitioning from the unconscious state of surgery to wakefulness in the recovery room, is managed carefully by the anaesthetic team. Anaesthetic agents are discontinued, and as their effects wear off over a period of minutes, consciousness gradually returns.

The breathing tube is typically removed once the patient is breathing adequately on their own and able to protect their airway, which usually occurs before or shortly after arrival in the recovery room. A sore throat, sometimes persisting for a day or two, is a common and temporary consequence of having had this tube in place during surgery.

Post-anaesthetic confusion or disorientation, sometimes called emergence delirium, can occur in the period immediately after waking, particularly in younger patients and older patients. This is typically brief, resolving over minutes to a couple of hours, and is managed by the recovery room nursing team with reassurance and a calm environment.

FROM THE SURGEON'S DESK

The anaesthetic team is, in many ways, the unsung partner in scoliosis surgery. While the surgical aspects of the procedure naturally attract most of the discussion, the anaesthetic management throughout a long, complex operation, involving major blood loss, specific positioning challenges, and the requirement to preserve neuromonitoring signal quality, is every bit as critical to the safety and success of the procedure.

I work closely with the same anaesthetic colleagues for the vast majority of my cases, and that continuity of working relationship, built over hundreds of shared procedures, is part of what allows complex cases to proceed smoothly and safely. When you ask about the experience of your surgical team, the anaesthetic team's experience in spinal deformity cases specifically is just as important a question as the surgeon's.

Chapter Twenty-Seven:

Special Considerations — Congenital And Neuromuscular Scoliosis

While much of this book has focused on the most common form of scoliosis, adolescent idiopathic scoliosis, patients and families dealing with congenital or neuromuscular scoliosis face additional considerations that warrant dedicated discussion. This chapter explores these specific situations in greater depth, recognising that the journey for these patients and families often involves additional layers of complexity beyond those covered in the general chapters of this book.

CONGENITAL SCOLIOSIS — A DIFFERENT STARTING POINT

As introduced in Chapter One, congenital scoliosis arises from abnormalities in vertebral formation during early fetal development. Unlike idiopathic scoliosis, where the bones themselves are normally formed but the overall alignment has deviated, congenital scoliosis involves the bones themselves being abnormally shaped or fused from birth.

The classification of congenital vertebral anomalies matters significantly for prognosis. A fully segmented hemivertebra, where the abnormal vertebra has normal growth plates on its own and is separate from the vertebrae above and below, tends to produce more progressive deformity because this abnormal vertebra continues to grow, contributing to ongoing curve progression. A non-segmented or incarcerated hemivertebra, where the abnormal vertebra is fused to adjacent vertebrae and has limited growth potential, tends to be more stable.

Unilateral bars, where multiple vertebrae are fused together on one side of the spine while normal growth continues on the opposite side, tend to produce particularly progressive and severe deformity because the imbalance between the growing and non-growing sides compounds over time.

Because of this variability, the management of congenital scoliosis is highly individualised, depending on the specific type of anomaly, its location, and the pattern of growth observed over time. Early and close monitoring, often beginning in infancy, is standard for congenital scoliosis, because the rate and pattern of progression in the first years of life provides crucial information for planning.

ASSOCIATED ANOMALIES IN CONGENITAL SCOLIOSIS

Because congenital scoliosis arises from disruptions during early fetal development, and because the development of the spine occurs alongside the development of other organ systems during the same embryonic period, congenital scoliosis is frequently associated with anomalies in other systems. This is sometimes referred to as the VACTERL association, an acronym describing a cluster of anomalies that can co-occur, including vertebral anomalies, anal anomalies, cardiac anomalies, tracheoesophageal anomalies, renal anomalies, and limb anomalies.

For this reason, patients diagnosed with congenital scoliosis typically undergo additional screening, including renal ultrasound to assess for kidney anomalies, cardiac assessment including echocardiography, and spinal MRI to assess for intraspinal anomalies such as a tethered spinal cord or syringomyelia, which occur with increased frequency in congenital scoliosis.

This additional screening is not intended to alarm families but reflects appropriate comprehensive care, ensuring that any associated conditions are identified and managed, and that the overall surgical planning accounts for the full picture of the child's anatomy and health.

SURGICAL APPROACHES IN CONGENITAL SCOLIOSIS

The surgical management of congenital scoliosis is highly individualised based on the specific anomaly, its location, the degree of deformity, and the age of the patient. Several specific surgical strategies are particularly relevant to congenital scoliosis.

Hemivertebra excision involves surgical removal of the abnormal vertebra itself, followed by fusion of the adjacent normal vertebrae to close the resulting gap and correct the deformity. This approach directly addresses the cause of the deformity and can be highly effective, particularly when performed at a younger age before significant secondary curvature has developed in the adjacent normal spine.

Convex growth arrest, sometimes called hemiepiphysiodesis, involves surgically halting growth on the convex (longer) side of the curve while allowing continued growth on the concave (shorter) side, gradually correcting the imbalance over time as the child grows. This approach is most effective in younger children with significant growth remaining and with curves that are not yet severe.

Growth-friendly strategies, including growing rods as discussed in Chapter Ten, may be used in congenital scoliosis to control the curve while preserving growth potential, particularly in younger children where definitive fusion would be premature.

NEUROMUSCULAR SCOLIOSIS — A COMPREHENSIVE CHALLENGE

Neuromuscular scoliosis, arising from underlying conditions including cerebral palsy, muscular dystrophy, spinal muscular atrophy, and others, presents a different set of challenges centred on the broader medical complexity of the patient and the specific characteristics of neuromuscular curves.

Neuromuscular curves tend to be larger, more rigid, and more likely to extend into the pelvis than idiopathic curves. Pelvic obliquity, meaning tilting of the pelvis as part of the overall spinal deformity, is common in neuromuscular scoliosis and has significant functional implications, particularly for seated positioning in patients who use wheelchairs.

The goals of surgery in neuromuscular scoliosis often differ in emphasis from idiopathic scoliosis. While correction of the deformity remains important, the functional goals often centre on improving seated balance and positioning, which has direct implications for comfort, skin integrity (reducing pressure sore risk from asymmetric seating), respiratory function, and the ability to use the upper limbs for daily activities without needing to use them for postural support.

MEDICAL COMPLEXITY AND PERIOPERATIVE PLANNING

Patients with neuromuscular scoliosis frequently have significant medical complexity beyond the spine itself, related to their underlying condition. This may include respiratory compromise related to the underlying neuromuscular condition itself, independent of the scoliosis, requiring careful pre-operative respiratory assessment and planning, including in some cases pre-operative initiation of non-invasive ventilation support. Nutritional considerations, as many patients with neuromuscular conditions have feeding difficulties and may require nutritional optimisation, sometimes including gastrostomy feeding, before major surgery. Cardiac involvement, particularly in certain forms of muscular dystrophy, requiring cardiac assessment as part of pre-operative planning. And seizure disorders, common in some neuromuscular conditions, requiring coordination of anti-seizure medication management around the surgical period.

The surgical team for neuromuscular scoliosis surgery is necessarily multidisciplinary, often involving the patient's neurologist, respiratory physician, and other specialists alongside the spinal surgical and anaesthetic teams, reflecting the comprehensive nature of care required.

OUTCOMES AND EXPECTATIONS IN NEUROMUSCULAR SCOLIOSIS

The outcomes of surgery for neuromuscular scoliosis are best understood within the context of the goals discussed above. Studies examining outcomes in this population, often using caregiver-reported outcome measures given the communication limitations some patients face, demonstrate improvements in seated positioning, ease of care including dressing and hygiene, comfort, and in some studies, respiratory function.

The complication rates in neuromuscular scoliosis surgery are generally higher than in idiopathic scoliosis surgery, reflecting both the greater complexity of the curves themselves and the broader medical complexity of the patient population. This is not a reason to avoid surgery when it is appropriately indicated, but it is a reason for thorough pre-operative discussion of realistic expectations and the specific risk profile for the individual patient.

FROM THE SURGEON'S DESK

Congenital and neuromuscular scoliosis represent some of the most complex cases I manage, and the families navigating these conditions are often already managing significant complexity in their lives before scoliosis surgery even becomes part of the picture.

What I try to do with these families is set goals collaboratively that reflect what matters most to them and to the patient, which may be quite different from the goals that would apply to an otherwise healthy adolescent with idiopathic scoliosis. For a child with severe cerebral palsy, improved seated comfort and easier caregiving may be the primary goals, and success looks different from the curve correction percentages that dominate discussions of idiopathic scoliosis outcomes.

These conversations require time, multidisciplinary input, and a willingness to define success in terms that are meaningful for each individual family's situation, not a one-size-fits-all framework borrowed from a different population of patients.

Chapter Twenty-Eight:

Travelling For Surgery And Navigating International Care

For some patients, accessing the most appropriate surgical expertise for their specific situation involves travelling, sometimes considerable distances, to reach a specialist centre. This chapter addresses the practical considerations involved in travelling for surgery, whether within your own country to a specialist centre, or internationally.

WHY PATIENTS TRAVEL FOR SCOLIOSIS SURGERY

As discussed extensively in Chapter Five, the experience and case volume of the surgical team and the comprehensiveness of the institutional resources, including intraoperative neuromonitoring, blood management, and post-operative care pathways, significantly influence outcomes in scoliosis surgery. In many regions, the concentration of this expertise is limited to a relatively small number of specialist centres, and patients living outside the immediate catchment area of these centres may need to travel to access them.

This is a normal and common aspect of accessing specialist surgical care for complex conditions, and the practical considerations involved are manageable with appropriate planning.

PRACTICAL CONSIDERATIONS FOR DOMESTIC TRAVEL TO A SPECIALIST CENTRE

When travelling within your own country to a specialist centre, several practical factors deserve attention. The pre-operative assessment process may require one or more visits to the specialist centre before the day of surgery itself, and understanding this schedule in advance allows for appropriate planning of time off work or school, and travel and accommodation arrangements for these visits.

Accommodation near the specialist centre, both for the pre-operative visits and particularly for the family during the hospital stay itself, should be arranged in advance. Many specialist hospitals have relationships with nearby accommodation providers, sometimes with discounted rates for patients' families, and the hospital's patient liaison or social work team can often provide guidance on this.

The discharge journey home requires specific consideration. Travelling home from the hospital after major spinal surgery, particularly if this involves a long car journey or other travel, needs to be planned with the surgical team's input regarding timing and any specific precautions, such as frequency of stops during a long car journey to allow position changes.

Follow-up care arrangements need to be considered from the outset. Some aspects of follow-up, including wound checks and suture removal, may be able to be managed locally by your own general practitioner or local hospital, with the specialist centre providing remote oversight, while other follow-up, particularly imaging review and milestone assessments, may require return visits to the specialist centre. Understanding this division of follow-up care in advance helps with planning.

INTERNATIONAL TRAVEL FOR SURGERY

For patients seeking surgery in a different country, whether because of the availability of specific expertise, healthcare system factors, or personal choice, additional considerations apply.

Medical record transfer is essential and should be arranged well in advance. This includes not just written reports but actual imaging files, which should ideally be provided in a standard digital format that can be reviewed by the receiving surgical team. Discuss with both your current and prospective surgical teams what specific records and images will be needed and how they should be transferred.

Communication and language considerations matter significantly for informed consent and for the quality of the doctor-patient relationship throughout the process. If there is a language difference between you and your surgical team, ensure that professional medical interpretation is available for all key consultations, rather than relying on informal translation, which can result in important information being missed or misunderstood.

Travel timing around surgery requires careful planning. Most surgical teams will advise against air travel for a defined period after major spinal surgery, often several weeks, due to the combination of prolonged sitting, the risk of deep vein thrombosis, and the physical demands of travel during early recovery. Planning for an extended stay in the location of surgery, sufficient to reach a stage of recovery where travel is considered safe, is an important practical and financial consideration.

Continuity of follow-up care after returning home requires explicit planning. Before travelling for surgery, discuss with the surgical team how follow-up will be managed once you return home: will this involve remote review of imaging obtained locally, periodic return visits, or transfer of ongoing care to a local specialist with the original surgical team available for consultation if needed. Having this plan in place before surgery, rather than figuring it out afterward, ensures continuity of the careful long-term follow-up that scoliosis surgery patients benefit from.

Insurance and financial planning for international medical travel involves understanding what costs are covered by your health insurance or the healthcare system arrangements of your home country, what additional costs (travel, accommodation, extended stay, potential complications requiring additional care) need to be planned for independently, and what arrangements exist for managing any complications that might occur after you have returned home, including whether the original surgical team can provide remote guidance to local healthcare providers if needed.

CULTURAL AND PRACTICAL CONSIDERATIONS

Patients and families travelling for surgery, whether domestically or internationally, are managing a major medical experience away from their normal support networks and familiar environment. This adds a layer of challenge to an already significant experience, and acknowledging this is important.

Bringing a support person, whether a family member or close friend, is valuable not only for the practical assistance they can provide but for the emotional support of having a familiar presence during an unfamiliar experience. If circumstances make this difficult, discuss with the receiving hospital what support resources, including patient liaison services, are available for patients without an accompanying support person.

Maintaining connection with home, through regular communication with family and friends, can provide important emotional support during what can be an isolating experience of being far from familiar surroundings during a vulnerable time.

FROM THE SURGEON'S DESK

I have operated on patients who have travelled significant distances, sometimes across continents, to reach our centre. Each time, I am struck by the additional layer of trust this represents: not only trusting a surgical team with a major operation, but doing so far from home, in an unfamiliar environment, often navigating language and cultural differences in addition to the medical experience itself.

For these patients and families, I try to be especially attentive to communication, ensuring that information is conveyed clearly and that there is ample opportunity for questions, recognising that the usual support networks that patients draw on, family doctors, local hospital staff they may know, are not as readily available. The practical planning discussed in this chapter, the medical record transfer, the follow-up arrangements, the support during the stay, all matter enormously for making this experience as smooth as possible for patients who have travelled to access the care they need.

CHAPTER TWENTY-NINE:

WHO'S WHO UNDERSTANDING YOUR MULTIDISCIPLINARY TEAM

Throughout this book, references have been made to many different professionals involved in scoliosis care: surgeons, anaesthetists, neurophysiologists, physiotherapists, and others. For patients and families navigating this process, encountering so many different professionals, often in quick succession during appointments and the hospital stay, can be disorienting. This chapter introduces each member of the team you are likely to encounter, explaining their specific role and how they contribute to your overall care.

THE SURGICAL TEAM

The lead surgeon is the consultant or attending spinal deformity surgeon who has overall responsibility for your surgical care, makes the key decisions about your surgical plan, and performs or directly supervises your operation. This is the person with whom you will have your primary consultations and who carries ultimate responsibility for your surgical journey.

Assistant surgeons, who may be more junior consultant colleagues, surgical fellows undergoing subspecialty training, or surgical trainees at various stages of their training, work alongside the lead surgeon during the operation, assisting with the procedure under the lead surgeon's supervision. Their involvement is a normal and important part of how complex surgery is performed at teaching hospitals, and it also reflects the training pathway through which future specialist surgeons develop their expertise.

THE ANAESTHETIC TEAM

The lead anaesthetist, often a consultant anaesthetist with specific experience in spinal deformity and neuroanaesthesia, is responsible for your safety and comfort throughout the anaesthetic, from the pre-operative assessment through the procedure itself and into the immediate recovery period. As discussed in Chapter Twenty-Six, this role requires specific expertise given the particular demands of scoliosis surgery anaesthesia.

Anaesthetic assistants, sometimes called anaesthetic nurses or anaesthetic technicians depending on the healthcare system, support the anaesthetist throughout the procedure, preparing equipment and medications and assisting with monitoring.

THE NEUROPHYSIOLOGY TEAM

The neurophysiologist, sometimes called an intraoperative neuromonitoring specialist, is responsible for setting up, conducting, and interpreting the continuous monitoring of your spinal cord and nerve root function throughout surgery, as discussed extensively in Chapter Nine. This specialist works in close communication with the surgical and anaesthetic teams throughout the procedure, providing the real-time safety information that is central to modern scoliosis surgery safety.

THE NURSING TEAM

Pre-operative nurses conduct your assessment before surgery, ensure all necessary preparations are complete, and prepare you for theatre.

Theatre nurses, including the scrub nurse who works directly with the surgical team handling instruments during the procedure, and the circulating nurse who manages the broader theatre environment, ensure that the operation proceeds smoothly from a nursing and logistical perspective.

Recovery room nurses care for you in the immediate post-anaesthetic period, monitoring your emergence from anaesthesia and managing your immediate post-operative needs as discussed in Chapter Eleven.

Ward nurses provide your ongoing care throughout your hospital stay, managing pain relief, monitoring your recovery, supporting your mobilisation, and being your primary point of contact for any concerns during your admission.

THE PHYSIOTHERAPY TEAM

Physiotherapists are central to your recovery from the first day after surgery through the months of rehabilitation. Inpatient physiotherapists work with you during your hospital stay, teaching safe movement techniques, supporting early mobilisation, and providing your initial home exercise programme. Outpatient physiotherapists continue your rehabilitation programme after discharge, progressing your exercises through the phases described in Chapter Fourteen and guiding your return to activity.

OTHER SPECIALISTS YOU MAY ENCOUNTER

Depending on your specific situation, additional specialists may be involved in your care. Radiologists are the specialist doctors who interpret your imaging studies, providing the reports that inform your surgical team's decisions, though you may not meet them directly as their role is largely behind the scenes. Haematologists may be involved in managing specific blood-related issues, particularly in patients with bleeding disorders or complex transfusion needs. Respiratory physicians may be involved in the assessment and management of patients with significant pulmonary involvement related to severe thoracic scoliosis. Dietitians may provide specific nutritional assessment and guidance, particularly for patients identified as having nutritional deficiencies or specific dietary needs. Psychologists or counsellors may be involved in providing the psychological support discussed throughout this book, particularly for patients experiencing significant anxiety or for whom the psychological dimensions of the surgical journey would benefit from specialist input. Social workers or patient liaison staff help coordinate the practical aspects of care, particularly for patients travelling for surgery as discussed in Chapter Twenty-Eight, or for families needing additional support resources.

ORTHOTISTS

For patients who have undergone bracing, as discussed in Chapter Twenty, the orthotist is the specialist responsible for designing, fitting, and adjusting the brace. While orthotists are most centrally involved in the pre-surgical phase for patients who brace, their role in the overall scoliosis care pathway is significant for many patients.

HOW THE TEAM WORKS TOGETHER

What may not be immediately visible to patients and families is the extent of communication and coordination that occurs among these team members, often outside of the appointments and interactions that patients directly observe. Multidisciplinary team meetings, where complex cases are discussed among relevant specialists before surgical planning is finalised, are standard practice at specialist centres. Pre-operative briefings, where the surgical and anaesthetic teams review the specific plan for each case before the day of surgery, ensure that everyone involved understands the plan and any specific considerations for that patient. Post-operative handovers, where information is communicated between the operating team and the ward team, and subsequently between shifts of ward staff, ensure continuity of care throughout your hospital stay.

FROM THE SURGEON'S DESK

One of the things I find most rewarding about working at a specialist centre is the team itself. Scoliosis surgery is fundamentally a team endeavour, and the quality of outcomes reflects not just my own technical ability but the collective expertise, communication, and coordination of everyone involved, from the neurophysiologist whose monitoring keeps the patient safe throughout the procedure, to the physiotherapist who will see the patient through months of recovery, to the ward nurse managing pain control on the second post-operative night.

When patients ask about their care team, I want them to understand that they are not simply under my care. They are under the care of a coordinated team of specialists, each contributing their specific expertise, working together toward the same outcome. Understanding who these people are and what they do is part of feeling oriented and informed throughout what can otherwise feel like an overwhelming number of new faces and roles.

CHAPTER THIRTY:

UNDERSTANDING COSTS, INSURANCE, AND HEALTHCARE SYSTEMS

The financial dimensions of major surgery vary enormously depending on the healthcare system within which a patient is being treated, and this chapter cannot provide specific financial guidance applicable to every reader's circumstances. What it can offer is a framework for understanding the types of costs involved in scoliosis surgery, the questions worth asking regardless of your healthcare system, and how to approach the financial planning aspects of this process.

CATEGORIES OF COST IN SCOLIOSIS SURGERY

Surgical and hospital fees represent the core cost of the procedure itself, including the surgical team's fees, the cost of the operating room time, the implants and instrumentation used, and the hospital stay. These costs can vary considerably depending on the complexity of the procedure, the length of fusion, and the specific implants used.

Anaesthetic fees cover the anaesthetic team's involvement throughout the procedure and may be billed separately from surgical fees in some healthcare systems.

Pre-operative assessment costs include the various tests and consultations described in Chapter Six: blood tests, imaging, anaesthetic consultation, and any specialist assessments required for your specific situation.

Post-operative care costs include the hospital stay itself, which can vary in length depending on your recovery, as well as ongoing outpatient follow-up appointments and physiotherapy sessions over the months following surgery.

Indirect costs, while not part of the medical bill itself, are an important part of the overall financial picture for many families. These include time off work for the patient and for caregivers, travel and accommodation costs particularly for patients travelling to specialist centres as discussed in Chapter Twenty-Eight, and the costs of home modifications and equipment discussed in Chapter Six.

NAVIGATING HEALTH INSURANCE

For patients with private health insurance, understanding your specific policy's coverage for scoliosis surgery is an important early step. Questions worth clarifying with your insurer include whether scoliosis surgery is covered under your policy, and if so, whether there are any waiting periods, exclusions, or pre-authorisation requirements that apply. What costs, if any, you will be responsible for, including deductibles, co-payments, or coverage limits. Whether your chosen surgeon and hospital are within your insurance network, and if not, what the financial implications of seeking care outside the network would be. Whether pre-authorisation or pre-certification is required before surgery can proceed, and what the process and timeline for this involves.

Obtaining clear, ideally written, confirmation of coverage before proceeding with surgery can prevent unexpected financial surprises and is worth the administrative effort it requires.

NAVIGATING PUBLICLY FUNDED HEALTHCARE SYSTEMS

For patients in countries with publicly funded healthcare systems, the financial considerations differ but planning remains important. Waiting times for scoliosis surgery within publicly funded systems can vary considerably, and understanding the expected timeline for your specific situation, including any factors that might affect prioritisation such as curve progression rate or symptom severity, helps with planning.

Some publicly funded systems include provisions for patients to seek care outside their immediate region, including in some cases internationally, if specific expertise is not available locally, with funding arrangements that vary by system. If your situation might benefit from this kind of arrangement, this is worth discussing explicitly with your treating team and the relevant administrative bodies within your healthcare system.

Indirect costs, including time off work, travel for appointments, and any equipment or home modifications, remain relevant considerations even within systems where the direct medical costs are publicly funded, and exploring what support, if any, exists for these costs within your specific system and circumstances is worthwhile.

QUESTIONS TO ASK ABOUT COSTS REGARDLESS OF YOUR SYSTEM

Whatever your healthcare system, several questions are universally useful to ask early in your surgical journey. What is the expected total cost of the procedure, including all components: surgical fees, hospital stay, anaesthetic fees, and implants. Are there any additional costs that might arise depending on how the surgery proceeds, such as the cost implications of an extended hospital stay if recovery is more complicated than typical, or the cost of any additional procedures that might be identified as necessary during surgery. What is covered by your insurance or healthcare system, and what, if anything, will you be responsible for directly. Is there a payment plan or financial counselling service available if direct costs are involved and represent a significant financial burden.

Many hospitals have financial counselling or patient liaison services specifically to help patients and families navigate these questions, and engaging with these services early in the process, well before the day of surgery, allows time to address any financial planning needs without this becoming an additional source of stress closer to the procedure itself.

THE VALUE PERSPECTIVE

While the financial aspects of major surgery are real and deserve careful attention, it is worth placing them in the context of the long-term value that successful scoliosis surgery provides, as documented throughout this book. The long-term outcome data discussed in Chapter Eighteen, the decades of improved quality of life, reduced pain, and restored function, represent a meaningful return on what is, for most patients, a significant but one-time investment, whether that investment is measured in direct financial terms, in the time and effort of the surgical journey, or both.

This is not to minimise the real financial pressures that many patients and families face, but rather to frame the decision within the fuller picture of what is being gained, alongside the costs involved in achieving it.

FROM THE SURGEON'S DESK

I am acutely aware that the financial dimensions of major surgery are a source of significant stress for many patients and families, on top of everything else this process involves. While the specifics of healthcare financing are largely outside my direct area of expertise, I try to ensure that patients and families have access to the people in our institution who can help navigate these questions: financial counsellors, patient liaison staff, and administrative teams experienced in working with insurers and healthcare funding bodies.

My strong advice is to engage with these resources early, well before the day of surgery, so that financial planning does not become an additional source of last-minute stress. The clinical team wants you focused on your physical and psychological preparation for surgery, not on unresolved financial questions that could have been addressed weeks earlier.

CHAPTER THIRTY-ONE:

THE FUTURE OF SCOLIOSIS CARE EMERGING RESEARCH AND DIRECTIONS

This book has focused primarily on established, evidence-based approaches to scoliosis diagnosis, treatment, and recovery. This final chapter looks ahead, exploring areas of active research and emerging developments that may shape the future of scoliosis care. While the content of this chapter is, by its nature, less settled than the rest of the book, understanding the directions of ongoing research provides useful context for patients, particularly those who may engage with scoliosis care, whether their own or a family member's, over many years.

GENETIC RESEARCH INTO IDIOPATHIC SCOLIOSIS

As discussed in Chapter One, the underlying cause of idiopathic scoliosis remains incompletely understood despite decades of research. Genetic research has identified numerous gene variants associated with increased risk of developing idiopathic scoliosis and with curve progression, though no single gene has been identified as a complete explanation, consistent with the likely multifactorial nature of the condition involving multiple genes interacting with growth and biomechanical factors.

The long-term aspiration of this research is the development of genetic risk profiling that could help identify, at an early stage, which patients with mild curves are at higher risk of progression and might benefit from earlier or more intensive monitoring or intervention, and conversely, which patients are at lower risk and might be appropriately managed with less intensive surveillance. While such tools are not yet part of routine clinical practice, the research in this area continues to advance.

ADVANCES IN VERTEBRAL BODY TETHERING AND GROWTH MODULATION

As discussed in Chapter Nine, vertebral body tethering represents a significant innovation in non-fusion surgical treatment for growing patients with idiopathic scoliosis. This remains an area of active research and refinement, with ongoing studies examining longer-term outcomes, refining patient selection criteria to better identify which patients are likely to achieve good results, and exploring technical refinements to the tethering technique itself, including tether materials and tensioning protocols.

As longer-term follow-up data from VBT cohorts accumulates, the role of this technique within the overall treatment landscape, including how it compares to traditional fusion for appropriately selected patients, will become increasingly well-defined.

ADVANCES IN SURGICAL NAVIGATION AND ROBOTICS

The trajectory of computer-assisted navigation and robotic surgical systems, discussed in Chapter Nine, continues to advance. Ongoing developments include further integration of navigation and robotic systems with intraoperative imaging, allowing real-time updates to the surgical plan as the procedure progresses and anatomy changes. Continued refinement of robotic systems toward greater autonomy in specific, well-defined surgical tasks, while surgical judgement and decision-making remain firmly with the surgical team. And the application of these technologies to an increasing range of spinal procedures and patient populations as the technology matures and becomes more widely available.

ADVANCES IN BIOLOGICAL FUSION ENHANCEMENT

Research into enhancing the biological process of bone fusion continues actively. This includes refinement of bone graft substitutes and biological agents that promote fusion, potentially reducing reliance on autologous bone graft harvest. Research into the biological mechanisms of non-union, with the goal of developing targeted interventions for patients at high risk of pseudarthrosis, such as those with specific metabolic risk factors. And exploration of biomaterials and implant coatings designed to enhance the integration between implants and surrounding bone, potentially improving the speed and reliability of fusion.

ARTIFICIAL INTELLIGENCE IN SCOLIOSIS CARE

The application of artificial intelligence and machine learning techniques to scoliosis care is an area of growing research interest. Potential applications include automated measurement of Cobb angles and other radiographic parameters from imaging, potentially improving consistency and efficiency of assessment. Predictive modelling to help identify which patients are at higher risk of curve progression, informing decisions about monitoring intensity and treatment timing. And surgical planning tools that use large datasets of previous cases to inform individualised predictions about expected correction and outcomes for a specific patient's anatomy.

As with any application of these technologies in healthcare, the integration of artificial intelligence tools into clinical practice requires careful validation, and these tools are generally understood as aids to clinical decision-making by experienced specialists, rather than replacements for that expertise.

LONG-TERM OUTCOME RESEARCH

As the cohorts of patients who underwent surgery with modern techniques, including pedicle screw instrumentation and routine intraoperative neuromonitoring, reach longer follow-up intervals, the evidence base regarding very long-term outcomes, beyond 20 and 30 years, continues to grow. This research will further refine our understanding of adjacent segment disease risk over the full lifespan, the long-term durability of modern instrumentation and fusion techniques, and the factors that predict the best long-term outcomes, informing increasingly individualised approaches to surgical planning.

A CLOSING PERSPECTIVE ON THE PACE OF PROGRESS

It is worth reflecting, in closing this chapter, on the pace of progress that has characterised scoliosis surgery over recent decades, as a basis for reasonable optimism about continued advancement. The introduction of segmental pedicle screw instrumentation transformed correction capability. The routine adoption of intraoperative neurophysiological monitoring transformed safety. The development of vertebral body tethering introduced a genuinely novel non-fusion option for appropriately selected growing patients. Each of these developments, now well-established parts of contemporary practice, represented significant advances when first introduced.

There is every reason to expect that the research directions outlined in this chapter, and others not yet conceived, will continue to refine and improve the care available to future patients, building on the substantial foundation of evidence and expertise that already exists.

FROM THE SURGEON'S DESK

I entered this field at a point in its development where many of the techniques I now consider routine were relatively new. Pedicle screw instrumentation throughout the thoracic spine, now standard, was still becoming established. Routine full-modality neuromonitoring, now non-negotiable, was earlier in its adoption. Vertebral body tethering did not exist as a clinical option.

I share this not to suggest that current practice is somehow provisional or incomplete, because the evidence behind current practice, as this book has documented extensively, is robust and the outcomes achievable today are genuinely excellent. But I share it because it gives me confidence that the trajectory of this field continues to point toward better outcomes, safer procedures, and more options for patients.

For a patient or family engaging with scoliosis care today, this means you are benefiting from decades of accumulated advancement, and the field continues to advance. That is a reasonable basis for confidence as you move forward with your own journey.

CHAPTER THIRTY-TWO:

FINAL THOUGHTS BRINGING IT ALL TOGETHER

This book has covered an enormous amount of ground: the anatomy of the spine, the nature of scoliosis in its various forms, the diagnostic journey, the decision to proceed with surgery, the surgical techniques themselves, the day of surgery, the recovery process in its phases, the risks and how they are managed, the long-term outcomes, and a wide range of practical and supportive topics for patients and families. This final chapter steps back to bring these threads together and to offer some closing perspective on how to approach the journey ahead.

THE THREAD THAT CONNECTS EVERYTHING

If there is a single thread that connects every chapter of this book, it is this: informed engagement improves outcomes. This is not a vague platitude but a conclusion supported by the evidence cited throughout these pages. Patients who understand their condition ask better questions and make more confident decisions. Patients who understand their surgery experience less pre-operative anxiety and report better post-operative pain control. Patients who understand their recovery engage more effectively with rehabilitation and achieve better functional outcomes. Patients who understand the warning signs to watch for access care more promptly when needed, improving outcomes in the rare situations where complications arise.

Every chapter of this book has been written in service of this single goal: to give you the understanding that translates into engaged, confident participation in your own care.

THE IMPORTANCE OF YOUR INDIVIDUAL JOURNEY

While this book has necessarily presented information in general terms, applicable to scoliosis patients broadly, your own journey is individual. Your specific curve, your specific health, your specific life circumstances, and your specific values and priorities all shape what the right path looks like for you.

This is why the relationship with your surgical team matters so much, and why the questions and checklists provided throughout this book are tools for that relationship rather than substitutes for it. The general evidence presented in these pages provides the foundation. Your surgical team's individualised application of that evidence to your specific situation is where the actual decisions about your care are made.

ON HOPE AND REALISM

Throughout this book, an effort has been made to balance hope with realism: to convey honestly that scoliosis surgery carries real risks and demands real commitment through a real recovery process, while also conveying honestly that the outcomes achievable, for the right patient with the right team, are genuinely excellent and consistently transformative.

Both halves of this balance matter. A purely hopeful account that minimised the challenges of surgery and recovery would leave patients unprepared for the reality they will experience, potentially undermining their confidence when that reality does not match an overly rosy picture. A purely cautionary account that emphasised only risks and challenges would fail to convey the genuine, evidence-based reasons for confidence that exist.

The truth, as is so often the case, lies in the full picture: real challenges, honestly presented, alongside real and substantial benefits, equally honestly presented, supported by decades of evidence from tens of thousands of patients.

A WORD ABOUT TIME

One theme that has recurred throughout this book is the role of time in scoliosis care. The diagnostic journey unfolds over months or years. The decision-making process deserves the time it needs. The surgery itself, while a single event, sits within a much longer arc of preparation beforehand and recovery afterward. The recovery itself unfolds over months, with fusion maturing over a year or more. And the long-term outcomes that this book has documented extend over decades.

Patience with this timeline, understanding that meaningful processes take the time they take, and that this is not a sign of anything going wrong but simply the nature of biological healing and adaptation, is one of the most valuable mindsets a patient can bring to this journey.

A WORD TO FAMILIES AND CAREGIVERS

This book has included a dedicated chapter for caregivers, but it is worth reiterating here, in these closing pages, that the journey through scoliosis surgery is rarely undertaken by a single person in isolation. Families navigate this together, and the support, practical and emotional, that family members and friends provide is woven throughout every stage of this process.

If you are a caregiver reading this book to support someone through their journey, your engagement matters. The understanding you build alongside the patient, the practical preparations you help make, and the emotional support you provide throughout, all contribute to the outcomes documented throughout this book.

A FINAL WORD

This book began with an author's note describing the questions that patients ask again and again in consultation rooms, and the desire to answer those questions fully, honestly, and in plain language. Having reached the end of this book, I hope those questions, and many others that arise along the way, feel more answerable than they did before.

Scoliosis surgery is a significant undertaking. It is also, for the right patient at the right time, performed by the right team, one of the most consistently transformative procedures in all of surgery. The evidence supports this. The decades of follow-up data support this. And the lives lived by patients after successful surgery, returning to the activities they love, standing differently in the world, free from the constant presence of a condition that had shaped the edges of their existence, support this.

Whatever stage of this journey you are at, whether you are just beginning to understand a recent diagnosis, preparing for surgery in the coming weeks, navigating the early days of recovery, or looking back on surgery from months or years down the line, I hope this book has served you well.

Thank you for reading. I wish you, or the person you are supporting, the very best outcome this journey can offer.

CHAPTER THIRTY-THREE:

ADULTS RETURNING TO SCOLIOSIS CARE AFTER DECADES

A significant and growing population of scoliosis patients are adults who were diagnosed in adolescence, perhaps treated with observation or bracing at the time, and who are now, decades later, returning to active scoliosis care because their curve has progressed and is now causing symptoms that affect their quality of life. This chapter is written specifically for this group of patients, who often arrive at a surgical consultation with a unique combination of familiarity with the condition and a sense of déjà vu about a decision they may have first encountered as teenagers.

THE EXPERIENCE OF RETURNING TO SCOLIOSIS CARE

For many adults in this situation, the experience of returning to active scoliosis discussions evokes memories, sometimes vivid, of their adolescent experience with the condition: the original diagnosis, perhaps a period of bracing, the X-rays, the appointments. These memories, whatever their emotional tone, shape how the adult patient approaches their current situation, sometimes in ways that are helpful and sometimes in ways that require updating.

One common experience is a sense that "nothing has changed" since adolescence, when in fact a great deal has changed, both in the patient's own curve, which has progressed over the decades, often accompanied by degenerative changes that were not present in adolescence, and in the field of scoliosis surgery itself, which has advanced substantially since the patient's adolescent experience, as discussed throughout this book.

Another common experience is carrying forward specific beliefs or fears from the adolescent experience, perhaps based on what was understood about scoliosis surgery decades ago, which may no longer accurately reflect contemporary practice. Patients whose adolescent understanding of scoliosis surgery involved longer hospital stays, less sophisticated instrumentation, the absence of routine intraoperative neuromonitoring, and less refined pain management protocols may carry forward an outdated picture of what surgery involves today.

WHY ADULT CURVES PROGRESS

As discussed in Chapter One, adult degenerative changes compound with pre-existing idiopathic curves in ways that can accelerate progression in adulthood, even for curves that were stable for years or decades after adolescence.

The mechanism involves the progressive degeneration of the intervertebral discs and facet joints that occurs with normal aging, occurring asymmetrically across an already-curved spine. Where a teenager's curve might have been relatively stable because the disc and joint structures, while curved, were healthy and symmetric in their load-bearing capacity, the same curve in a 50 or 60-year-old spine is subject to asymmetric degenerative changes that can accelerate the progression of the existing curve, sometimes substantially, over a relatively short period in mid-to-late adulthood.

This is why patients who were told as teenagers that their curve "didn't need surgery" and who experienced decades of stability may suddenly find, in their 40s, 50s, or 60s, that their curve is progressing more rapidly and causing new or worsening symptoms.

THE DIFFERENT SYMPTOM PROFILE IN ADULT PRESENTATION

Adults returning to scoliosis care often present with a different symptom profile than adolescents. While adolescents may have minimal symptoms beyond the visible deformity itself, adults frequently present with back pain, which is often the dominant symptom and may be the primary reason for seeking medical attention. Radicular symptoms, meaning pain, numbness, or weakness radiating into the legs, related to nerve root compression from the combination of deformity and degenerative stenosis. Neurogenic claudication, meaning leg pain, weakness, or heaviness brought on by walking or standing and relieved by sitting or bending forward, related to spinal stenosis.

And progressive functional limitation, including difficulty with activities that were previously straightforward, and in more severe cases, difficulty maintaining an upright posture for extended periods.

This different symptom profile means that the surgical indications and goals for adult patients, as discussed in Chapter Ten, are often more directly tied to symptom relief than the primarily deformity-correction-focused goals of adolescent surgery, though deformity correction, particularly sagittal balance restoration, remains centrally important to achieving good symptomatic outcomes.

THE COMPLEXITY OF ADULT SURGICAL PLANNING

As discussed extensively in Chapter Ten, adult scoliosis surgery is substantially more complex than adolescent surgery, and this complexity is often most apparent in patients returning to care after decades, where the combination of the original idiopathic curve and subsequent degenerative changes can create a particularly intricate surgical picture.

The surgical plan for these patients often needs to address multiple issues simultaneously: the original coronal deformity, sagittal plane changes that may have developed over the decades, stenosis at one or more levels causing neurological symptoms, and the overall balance of the spine in three dimensions. This often results in more extensive surgical plans than these patients may have anticipated based on their adolescent experience, when a more limited fusion might have been discussed.

UNDERSTANDING WHY "MORE SURGERY THAN EXPECTED" MAY BE RECOMMENDED

Patients returning to scoliosis care after decades sometimes find that the surgical plan recommended is more extensive than what they recall being discussed in adolescence, and this can be a source of concern or confusion. Understanding why this is the case, rather than experiencing it as an unexplained escalation, is valuable.

The curve itself has likely changed. Decades of progression mean the curve being addressed now is different, often larger and more complex, than the curve that might have been discussed in adolescence. Additional pathology has developed. The degenerative changes discussed above, including stenosis and disc degeneration at multiple levels, represent additional problems that need to be addressed, beyond the original deformity alone. The goals have shifted. Where an adolescent surgical plan might focus primarily on correcting a structural curve in an otherwise healthy spine, an adult surgical plan must also address symptom relief, neurological decompression, and the restoration of sagittal balance, each of which may require additional surgical steps including osteotomies and decompression procedures at multiple levels.

This is not "more surgery for the sake of it." It reflects the surgical plan needed to address the actual clinical picture as it exists now, which is different from the clinical picture that existed decades ago.

EMOTIONAL CONSIDERATIONS FOR THIS PATIENT GROUP

Adults returning to scoliosis care after decades sometimes carry complex emotions about this return: a sense of "having to deal with this again," frustration that a condition managed in adolescence has resurfaced as a significant issue in adulthood, and sometimes a sense of having "failed" to avoid surgery that was perhaps hoped to have been avoided permanently after adolescence.

These feelings are understandable and worth acknowledging. It is also worth reframing them where possible: the adolescent decision, whatever it was, was appropriate based on the information and curve characteristics at that time. The current situation reflects new information, a curve and clinical picture that have evolved over decades, and a decision-making process that, just as in adolescence, is based on the evidence and circumstances as they currently exist. There is no failure in this. There is simply the natural evolution of a condition over a lifetime, being addressed appropriately at each stage with the information and tools available.

FROM THE SURGEON'S DESK

I see many patients in this situation, adults in their 40s, 50s, and 60s, who were diagnosed with scoliosis as teenagers and are now, decades later, facing surgery for the first time. The conversations with these patients often have a particular quality, a blend of familiarity with the broad concept of scoliosis and surprise at how much has changed, both in their own spine and in the field of surgery itself.

I try to explicitly bridge this gap: acknowledging what they remember from their adolescent experience, explaining how their current situation differs from and builds on that earlier picture, and updating their understanding of what contemporary scoliosis surgery involves, much of which, as this book has documented throughout, has advanced substantially since their adolescent encounters with the condition.

For these patients, much of the value of a book like this one lies in updating decades-old understanding with current evidence, current techniques, and current outcomes, providing the same foundation of informed engagement that this book aims to provide for patients of any age and at any stage of their scoliosis journey.

CHAPTER THIRTY-FOUR:

HOW SURGEONS DECIDE WHICH LEVELS TO FUSE

One of the most technically important, and to patients often most opaque, decisions in scoliosis surgery is the determination of exactly which vertebral levels will be included in the fusion. This chapter aims to demystify this decision-making process, explaining the principles that guide it and why the answer is rarely as simple as "fuse the curved part."

THE FUNDAMENTAL PRINCIPLE — FUSE WHAT IS NECESSARY, PRESERVE WHAT IS POSSIBLE

The foundational principle of fusion level selection, referenced throughout this book, is to include the minimum number of vertebral levels necessary to achieve a stable, balanced correction, while preserving as many mobile, unfused segments as possible. Every level included in the fusion contributes to the correction and stability of the construct, but also represents motion that is permanently sacrificed and load that is transferred to the adjacent unfused segments.

This principle sounds straightforward, but applying it to an individual patient's specific curve pattern requires consideration of multiple interacting factors.

DETERMINING THE UPPER AND LOWER INSTRUMENTED VERTEBRAE

The upper instrumented vertebra and the lower instrumented vertebra define the extent of the fusion: the topmost and bottommost vertebrae that will be included in the instrumented construct. Selecting these levels appropriately is central to achieving a balanced, stable result.

For the lower instrumented vertebra, several specific considerations guide selection. The stable vertebra is the lowest vertebra that is bisected by a vertical line drawn from the centre of the sacrum on a standing X-ray. Ending the fusion at or near this level helps ensure the fusion ends on a vertebra that is centred over the pelvis, supporting overall balance. The neutral vertebra is the lowest vertebra that shows minimal rotation on the X-ray, indicating it is not significantly involved in the structural curve. Ending the fusion at a level where rotation has substantially resolved reduces the risk of the fusion ending within the structural curve itself, which could result in residual imbalance.

Fusing too short, meaning ending the lower instrumented vertebra within the structural curve or above the stable vertebra, risks leaving residual coronal imbalance, where the trunk remains shifted to one side, or progressive curvature below the fusion in the unfused segments, sometimes called "adding on," where the curve effectively continues below the fusion over time.

Fusing too long, extending the lower instrumented vertebra further into the lumbar spine than necessary, sacrifices additional lumbar motion segments, which, as discussed in Chapter Fourteen, has implications for long-term flexibility and may increase the biomechanical demand on the segments below the fusion, potentially increasing adjacent segment disease risk at the lumbosacral junction, a particularly important and mobile region.

For the upper instrumented vertebra, the considerations relate to the overall shape of the spine above the fusion and the biomechanics of the cervicothoracic and upper thoracic junction. Selecting an upper instrumented vertebra that results in a smooth transition to the unfused spine above, without creating an abrupt change in alignment that could predispose to proximal junctional kyphosis as discussed in Chapter Fifteen, is an important consideration.

SELECTIVE THORACIC FUSION

In certain curve patterns, particularly where there is a structural thoracic curve and a smaller, more flexible lumbar curve, a strategy called selective thoracic fusion may be appropriate: fusing the thoracic curve while leaving the lumbar curve unfused, on the basis that the lumbar curve, being more flexible, will spontaneously improve once the thoracic curve above it is corrected and the overall spinal balance is restored.

This strategy, when appropriate, preserves valuable lumbar motion segments. However, selecting patients appropriately for selective thoracic fusion requires careful pre-operative assessment of curve flexibility, as discussed in Chapter Three, because performing a selective fusion in a patient whose lumbar curve is more structural than initially assessed can result in residual imbalance requiring the lumbar curve to also be addressed, sometimes in a subsequent procedure.

THE ROLE OF SAGITTAL PLANE CONSIDERATIONS

As emphasised throughout this book, particularly in the context of adult deformity surgery, sagittal balance is a critical determinant of outcomes. Fusion level selection must account for the sagittal profile of the spine, not just the coronal curve.

In adolescent idiopathic scoliosis, this typically means ensuring that the fusion preserves or restores normal thoracic kyphosis and lumbar lordosis, avoiding either flattening the spine, which can predispose to sagittal imbalance and pain, or creating excessive curvature.

In adult deformity surgery, sagittal plane considerations often dominate the fusion level decision. The lower instrumented vertebra in adult deformity surgery is frequently extended to the sacrum or pelvis, a decision with significant implications for biomechanics and for long-term outcomes, made when the lumbosacral junction itself is a source of pathology, such as significant degeneration or instability at this level, that needs to be directly addressed as part of the overall correction.

WHY YOUR SPECIFIC FUSION LEVELS MATTER TO YOU

Understanding the fusion levels recommended for your specific case, and the reasoning behind them, is valuable for several reasons beyond simple curiosity.

It helps you understand the functional implications discussed in Chapter Fourteen: which regions of your spine will retain mobility and which will not, informing realistic expectations about flexibility after surgery.

It provides context for any future imaging or assessments: knowing your fusion levels allows you to understand references to "the upper instrumented vertebra" or "the level above the fusion" in future reports or discussions.

And it can be relevant if you experience symptoms in the future: understanding which segments are fused and which are not helps frame discussions about whether new symptoms relate to the fused construct, to adjacent unfused segments, or to an entirely separate issue.

FROM THE SURGEON'S DESK

Fusion level selection is, in many ways, the most intellectually demanding part of pre-operative planning for scoliosis surgery. It requires synthesising information about the curve's structure, flexibility, and rotation, the patient's overall spinal balance in both the coronal and sagittal planes, and an understanding of how the proposed construct will behave not just immediately after surgery but over the decades that follow.

I spend considerable time on this aspect of planning for every patient, often reviewing the imaging multiple times, considering different scenarios, and in complex cases, discussing the plan with colleagues before finalising it. When I explain the fusion levels to a patient, I am sharing the outcome of that careful planning process, and I am always happy to walk through the reasoning in more detail for patients who want to understand it. It is, after all, their spine, and their long-term outcome that this planning is designed to optimise.

CHAPTER THIRTY-FIVE:

A CLOSER LOOK AT POST-OPERATIVE EXERCISES

Chapter Fourteen described the phases of rehabilitation in general terms. This chapter provides more specific descriptions of the types of exercises typically included at each phase, giving patients a clearer picture of what physiotherapy sessions and home exercise programmes are likely to involve. As always, the specific exercises appropriate for you should be determined by your own physiotherapy team based on your individual surgery and recovery, and this chapter is intended to provide context and understanding rather than a programme to follow independently.

PHASE ONE EXERCISES — THE FOUNDATION

Diaphragmatic breathing exercises involve lying or sitting comfortably and breathing deeply, focusing on expanding the lower ribs and abdomen rather than the upper chest, holding briefly, and exhaling slowly. These exercises, performed for several minutes multiple times daily, support full lung expansion and help prevent the small areas of lung collapse that can occur after surgery, particularly relevant after thoracic procedures.

Ankle pumps and circles involve moving the feet up and down at the ankle, and rotating the feet in circles, performed regularly while resting in bed or sitting. These simple movements promote circulation in the legs and are an important part of reducing blood clot risk in the early post-operative period.

The log roll technique, while not an exercise in the traditional sense, is a movement pattern that is practised repeatedly in the early days, as described in Chapter Twelve: rolling onto the side as a unit, using the arms to push to a seated position while the legs move together over the edge of the bed, avoiding any bending or twisting of the spine during the transition from lying to sitting.

Walking, the centrepiece of phase one as discussed extensively in Chapter Thirteen, begins as short distances around the room or ward and progressively increases. While walking is an activity rather than a discrete exercise, the way it is performed matters: an upright posture, looking ahead rather than down, and a normal walking pattern without excessive caution or altered gait, to the extent pain allows, supports the most efficient recovery of normal movement patterns.

Gentle shoulder and arm movements, including shoulder rolls and arm raises performed within a comfortable range, help maintain upper body mobility and can relieve some of the muscular tension that develops in the shoulders and upper back during the prone positioning of surgery and the restricted movement of early recovery.

PHASE TWO EXERCISES — BUILDING THE FOUNDATION

Transversus abdominis activation, often introduced as one of the first specific core exercises, involves lying on the back with knees bent, and gently drawing the lower abdomen in and up, as though drawing the navel toward the spine, without holding the breath or tensing the larger superficial abdominal muscles. This subtle activation of the deep abdominal wall is held for several seconds and repeated, gradually building the capacity of this important stabilising muscle.

Pelvic tilts involve lying on the back with knees bent, and gently flattening the lower back against the floor or bed by tilting the pelvis, then releasing back to neutral. This gentle movement helps restore awareness and control of lumbar spine positioning.

Heel slides involve lying on the back with knees bent, and slowly sliding one heel away along the floor to straighten the leg, then sliding it back, while maintaining the core activation and a stable spine position. This exercise begins to introduce controlled lower limb movement while challenging the core stabilisers to maintain spinal position.

Bridging, introduced when appropriate for the individual's recovery stage, involves lying on the back with knees bent and feet flat, and gently lifting the hips off the bed or floor by squeezing the buttocks and pushing through the feet, then lowering slowly. This exercise builds strength in the gluteal muscles and provides a controlled loading of the lower back and hip extensors.

Standing balance exercises, including standing on one leg with support as needed, begin to challenge the proprioceptive and balance systems that contribute to overall functional stability.

Gentle hip flexor and hamstring stretches, performed within a comfortable range and without bouncing or forcing, address the tightness that commonly develops in these muscle groups during the restricted movement of early recovery.

PHASE THREE EXERCISES — EXPANDING CAPACITY

Progressive resistance exercises for the major muscle groups, introduced under physiotherapy guidance, build overall strength in a way that supports the spine and the activities of daily life. These might include modified squats, performed with attention to maintaining a neutral spine position throughout the movement, leg press or similar machine-based exercises that allow controlled, progressive loading without the spinal demands of free-weight exercises, and upper body exercises addressing the muscles of the back, shoulders, and arms.

Functional movement training addresses the specific movement patterns required for daily activities and, where relevant, return to sport. This might include practising safe lifting techniques, hinging at the hips with a stable spine, practising stepping and turning patterns relevant to daily mobility, and for patients returning to specific sports, sport-specific movement patterns introduced progressively under guidance.

Cardiovascular conditioning exercises, including walking at increasing pace and distance, stationary cycling at increasing resistance and duration, and swimming with an increasing range of strokes as cleared, build the overall fitness that supports both general health and the capacity for the physical activities the patient wishes to return to.

Balance and proprioception exercises, building on the foundations introduced in phase two, become more challenging, potentially including exercises on unstable surfaces under appropriate supervision, supporting the coordination and stability needed for a confident return to varied activities.

THE IMPORTANCE OF INDIVIDUALISATION

While this chapter has described general categories of exercises typical at each phase, the specific exercise programme for any individual patient should be developed and progressed by their own physiotherapy team, taking into account the specific extent of their surgery, their individual recovery progress, any complications or specific considerations, and their personal goals for return to activity.

Patients sometimes encounter exercise information from sources other than their own physiotherapy team, whether from books like this one, from online sources, or from well-meaning friends and family who have had different experiences. While general understanding of the categories and progression of post-operative exercise, as provided in this chapter, is valuable, the specific application to your own recovery should always be guided by your own treating physiotherapist, who has direct knowledge of your surgery and ongoing assessment of your recovery.

FROM THE SURGEON'S DESK

I have enormous respect for the physiotherapists I work with, whose expertise in translating the surgical correction into functional recovery is, in many ways, as important to the ultimate outcome as the surgery itself.

What I want patients to take from this chapter is a sense of the progression involved: from the simple, almost deceptively basic movements of phase one, breathing, ankle pumps, careful transfers, through the building work of phase two's core stabilisation, to the genuinely athletic conditioning of phase three for patients working toward a full return to sport or demanding activity.

Each phase builds on the last. There are no shortcuts that skip phases, because each phase establishes the physiological and functional foundation that the next phase builds upon. Patience with this progression, and trust in the expertise of the physiotherapy team guiding it, are among the most valuable things a patient can bring to their rehabilitation.

Appendix A

GLOSSARY OF TERMS

APPENDIX: GLOSSARY OF TERMS

Adjacent segment disease: Degenerative changes developing in the spinal levels immediately above or below a spinal fusion, related to the increased mechanical load these levels bear when the fused segments cannot contribute to normal spinal motion.

Adolescent idiopathic scoliosis (AIS): The most common form of scoliosis, developing in otherwise healthy adolescents between approximately ages 10 and 18, with no identifiable underlying cause. More likely to progress to surgical thresholds in girls than in boys.

Allograft: Bone graft material derived from a human donor through a bone bank. Provides osteoconductive scaffold to supplement patient autograft in spinal fusion.

Annulus fibrosus: The tough outer fibrous ring of an intervertebral disc, composed of multiple concentric fibrocartilaginous layers providing tensile strength and containing the nucleus pulposus.

Anterior approach: Surgical access to the spine from the front of the body. In the thoracic spine via thoracotomy; in the lumbar spine via a retroperitoneal approach.

Articular processes: Bony projections on each vertebra that form facet joints with adjacent vertebrae. Superior articular processes face upward; inferior articular processes face downward.

Atlas: The first cervical vertebra (C1), ring-shaped, which supports the skull and articulates with the axis below.

Autograft: Bone graft taken from the patient's own body. Gold standard for spinal fusion because it contains osteogenic cells, osteoinductive growth factors, and osteoconductive scaffold simultaneously.

Axis: The second cervical vertebra (C2), which has the dens projection allowing rotational movement of the atlas and skull above.

Bone morphogenetic protein (BMP): A biologically active protein that powerfully stimulates bone formation. Recombinant human BMP-2 is used as a fusion adjunct in high-risk patients.

Cancellous bone: The porous inner bone tissue within vertebral bodies, less dense than cortical bone but well-vascularised and metabolically active, making it an important component of autograft.

Cauda equina: The bundle of nerve roots descending from the end of the spinal cord (approximately L1/L2) through the lumbar canal to their exit levels. Supplies lower limbs, bladder, bowel, and genitals.

Cell salvage: Intraoperative collection, processing, and re-infusion of shed blood, returning a significant proportion of surgical blood loss to the patient as transfusable autologous red cells.

Cervical spine: The uppermost mobile spinal region, comprising seven vertebrae (C1 to C7) in the neck. Greatest range of motion of any spinal region.

Cobb angle: The standardised measurement of scoliosis severity in degrees, measured on standing full-length X-ray as the angle between lines along the superior endplate of the upper end vertebra and the inferior endplate of the lower end vertebra.

Congenital scoliosis: Scoliosis caused by abnormalities in vertebral formation during fetal development, including hemivertebra and block vertebra.

Coronal balance: Side-to-side spinal alignment assessed on frontal standing X-ray. A plumb line from C7 should pass through the sacral midline in a well-balanced spine.

Cortical bone: The dense, hard outer shell of bone forming the boundary of vertebral bodies and all bony structures.

Degenerative scoliosis: Also called de novo adult scoliosis. Lateral curvature developing in adults from asymmetric disc degeneration and facet joint arthritis, predominantly in the lumbar spine.

Decortication: Surgical removal of the outer cortical bone layer from posterior spinal elements during fusion bed preparation, exposing vascular cancellous bone to promote graft incorporation.

DEXA scan: Dual-energy X-ray absorptiometry. The standard method for measuring bone mineral density and assessing osteoporosis.

Dura mater: The tough outer membrane enclosing the spinal cord, nerve roots, and cerebrospinal fluid. Inadvertent surgical entry causes a dural tear and CSF leak.

End vertebra: The most tilted vertebra at the top or bottom of a scoliotic curve, used as the reference point for Cobb angle measurement.

Facet joints: Small paired synovial joints at the posterior of each vertebral level, formed by articular processes of adjacent vertebrae. Guide spinal motion and provide rotational stability. Also called zygapophyseal joints.

Foramen (foramina): Openings in the spinal column through which nerve roots exit the canal at each vertebral level. Stenosis of these openings causes nerve root compression.

Growing rods: Implants used in early onset scoliosis to control curve progression while allowing continued spinal growth, periodically lengthened either surgically or by an external magnet.

Hemivertebra: A congenitally incomplete vertebra, present on only one side, creating a wedge that tilts the spine above it.

Hueter-Volkmann law: The principle that compression slows growth plate growth while tension accelerates it. The biological basis for vertebral body tethering.

Idiopathic: Of unknown cause. Applied to the most common form of scoliosis where the specific causative mechanism has not been identified.

Iliac crest: The curved upper border of the ilium forming the prominent hip bone. The iliac apophysis along this border provides the Risser sign.

Instrumentation: The collective metal hardware of spinal surgery including pedicle screws, connecting rods, hooks, wires, and cross-connectors.

Intervertebral disc: The fibrocartilaginous cushion between adjacent vertebral bodies consisting of the outer annulus fibrosus and inner nucleus pulposus. Functions as shock absorber, spacer, and flexible joint.

Intraoperative neurophysiological monitoring (IONM): Continuous real-time monitoring of spinal cord and nerve root function during surgery using SSEP and MEP signals.

Kyphosis: Forward-bending sagittal curvature. Normal in the thoracic spine. Abnormal when excessive, causing a rounded back deformity.

Lamina (laminae): Flat bony plates forming the posterior arch of each vertebra, constituting the back wall of the spinal canal.

Lateral approach: Surgical access to the lumbar spine through the patient's flank, used in XLIF and LLIF procedures to reach the disc space from the side.

Ligamentum flavum: Paired elastic ligament connecting adjacent laminae, forming part of the spinal canal back wall. Can thicken with age and contribute to stenosis.

Lordosis: Backward-bending sagittal curvature. Normal in the cervical and lumbar spine, providing the characteristic inward curves of these regions.

Lumbar spine: The lower mobile spinal region comprising five vertebrae (L1 to L5). Bears the greatest compressive load and provides most forward-bending motion.

Magnetically controlled growing rod: A growing rod device with an internal motor that can be lengthened non-invasively by an external magnet in clinic, avoiding repeated surgical procedures for lengthening.

Motor evoked potentials (MEPs): Intraoperative monitoring signals generated by transcranial brain stimulation, recording muscle responses in the legs to test motor pathway integrity through the spinal cord.

Multifidus: Deep paraspinal muscle critical for dynamic spinal stabilisation. Specifically targeted in post-operative rehabilitation for core stabilisation.

Neuromuscular scoliosis: Scoliosis resulting from an underlying neurological or muscular condition causing muscle weakness or imbalance around the spine.

Non-union (pseudarthrosis): Failure of bone graft to form solid continuous bone across one or more fusion segments, leaving those segments without biological support for the instrumentation.

Nucleus pulposus: The gel-like central core of the intervertebral disc with high water content, providing hydraulic cushioning and load distribution.

Osteoconductive: Property of bone graft material providing a physical scaffold for new bone growth.

Osteogenic: Property of bone graft material relating to the presence of viable bone-forming cells within the graft.

Osteoinductive: Property of bone graft material relating to chemical signals that stimulate surrounding cells to become bone-forming cells.

Osteotomy: Controlled surgical bone cut used in spinal deformity surgery to allow vertebral segment repositioning and achieve correction not possible through instrumentation alone.

Osteoporosis: Reduced bone mineral density causing fragility and compromising pedicle screw purchase.

Paraspinal muscles: Muscle groups running along both sides of the spine from pelvis to skull, responsible for spinal movement and postural support.

Pedicle: Short, stout bony bridge connecting the vertebral body to the posterior vertebral elements. Entry point and channel for pedicle screws.

Pedicle screw: Titanium screw placed through the pedicle into the vertebral body, providing the primary fixation point for connecting rods in modern spinal instrumentation.

Pedicle subtraction osteotomy: Surgical removal of posterior elements, pedicles, and a vertebral body wedge to allow approximately 30 to 40 degrees of sagittal correction at a single level.

Posterior approach: Surgical access to the spine from the patient's back. The most commonly used approach for scoliosis correction.

Proximal junctional kyphosis (PJK): Forward bending deformity developing in the spinal levels immediately above the upper end of a spinal fusion.

Risser sign: Measure of skeletal maturity graded 0 to 5 based on ossification of the iliac apophysis along the iliac crest, visible on standard spinal X-ray.

Rod: Connecting bar (titanium or cobalt-chromium alloy) linking pedicle screws in spinal instrumentation, transmitting corrective and stabilising forces between fixation points.

Sacrum: Triangular fused bone at the spine base, connecting the spinal column to the pelvis.

Sagittal balance: Front-to-back spinal alignment assessed on lateral standing X-ray. The most important predictor of functional outcomes after adult spinal deformity surgery.

Scoliosis Research Society (SRS): The primary international professional organisation for spinal deformity specialists, establishing clinical guidelines and collecting outcome data.

Somatosensory evoked potentials (SSEPs): Intraoperative monitoring signals generated by peripheral nerve stimulation and recorded at the brain, testing sensory pathway integrity through the spinal cord.

Spinal canal: The bony tunnel through which the spinal cord travels, formed by the vertebral bodies anteriorly and the neural arches posteriorly.

Spinal cord: The main neural structure within the spinal canal, carrying motor and sensory signals between brain and body. Ends at approximately L1 to L2 in adults.

Spinal stenosis: Narrowing of the spinal canal or intervertebral foramina causing neural compression.

Spinous process: Posterior bony projection from the laminar junction, palpable as the midline bumps of the back.

Syringomyelia: A fluid-filled cavity within the spinal cord, associated with atypical scoliosis patterns and identifiable on MRI.

Thoracic insufficiency syndrome: Inability of the thoracic cage to support normal breathing due to impaired thoracic growth, a risk of early rigid spinal fusion in young children.

Thoracic spine: The middle spinal region comprising 12 vertebrae (T1 to T12), each articulating with a rib pair.

Thoracoscopy: Minimally invasive chest surgery using ports and a camera, avoiding open thoracotomy for access to the thoracic spine.

Thoracotomy: Open surgical incision through the chest wall providing direct access to the thoracic spine for anterior approaches.

Transverse process: Lateral bony projections at the pedicle-lamina junction serving as muscle and ligament attachment points and rib articulation sites in the thoracic spine.

Vertebra: An individual bone of the spinal column. Plural: vertebrae.

Vertebral body: The large anterior cylindrical bone component of each vertebra, bearing the primary compressive load of the spine.

Vertebral body tethering (VBT): Non-fusion surgical technique for adolescent scoliosis using a flexible cord on the convex curve side to modulate differential growth and correct the deformity without fusion.

XLIF and LLIF: Extreme Lateral Interbody Fusion and Lateral Lumbar Interbody Fusion. Minimally invasive lateral approaches to the lumbar spine for disc removal and cage placement, avoiding open posterior muscle dissection.

Zygapophyseal joints: Another term for facet joints, the small paired posterior synovial joints at each vertebral level.

APPENDIX B

This appendix provides an overview of the types of research and resources that inform the content of this book, along with guidance on how patients can engage with the medical literature if they wish to explore topics in greater depth.

UNDERSTANDING THE EVIDENCE BASE

The information in this book is drawn from several categories of evidence that form the foundation of modern scoliosis care.

Randomised controlled trials represent the highest level of evidence in clinical research, comparing two or more treatment approaches in groups of patients randomly assigned to each, minimising the influence of other factors on the observed outcomes. The BrAIST trial, discussed in detail in Chapter Twenty, is a landmark example in scoliosis care, providing definitive evidence for the effectiveness of bracing.

Large cohort studies follow groups of patients over time, often for decades, documenting outcomes and identifying factors associated with better or worse results. Much of the long-term outcome data discussed in Chapter Eighteen comes from such studies, some following patients for 20 to 25 years after adolescent idiopathic scoliosis surgery.

Clinical practice guidelines synthesise the available evidence into recommendations for practice, developed by expert panels including organisations such as the Scoliosis Research Society. These guidelines represent the consensus of the field on best practice, while acknowledging areas of ongoing uncertainty.

Case series and registry data provide information on outcomes and complication rates from large numbers of patients treated at specific institutions or across networks of institutions, contributing to our understanding of real-world outcomes beyond the controlled conditions of clinical trials.

KEY ORGANISATIONS AND RESOURCES

The Scoliosis Research Society is the major international professional organisation dedicated to the study and treatment of spinal deformities. It publishes patient information resources, supports research, and establishes practice guidelines that inform care at specialist centres worldwide.

National and regional scoliosis support organisations exist in many countries, providing patient information, support networks, and advocacy. These organisations can be valuable sources of practical information and peer support, complementing the medical information provided by your surgical team.

Hospital-based patient education programmes, where available, provide structured information sessions, often including the opportunity to meet other patients and families navigating similar experiences, and to ask questions in a less time-pressured environment than a clinical consultation.

ENGAGING WITH MEDICAL LITERATURE AS A PATIENT

For patients who wish to explore the research literature directly, several principles can help navigate this material productively. Peer-reviewed journals, where articles have been reviewed by independent experts before publication, provide more reliable information than non-peer-reviewed sources. Look for studies with larger numbers of patients and longer follow-up periods, as these generally provide more reliable information than small or short-term studies. Be cautious of individual case reports or testimonials, which describe single experiences that may not be representative of typical outcomes.

When in doubt about how a particular piece of research applies to your individual situation, discuss it with your surgical team. They can help contextualise research findings within the framework of your specific diagnosis and circumstances.

A NOTE ON MEDICAL INFORMATION ONLINE

The internet contains an enormous volume of information about scoliosis, of widely varying quality and accuracy. As discussed in Chapter One, online forums and discussion groups can be valuable for peer support but can also contain information that is outdated, based on individual anecdote rather than evidence, or simply incorrect.

When evaluating online medical information, consider the source: information from established medical institutions, professional societies, and government health agencies generally reflects a higher standard of accuracy than information from individual blogs, forums, or commercial sites with a product to sell. Be alert to claims that seem too certain, too simple, or too good to be true, as medicine rarely deals in such absolutes. And always bring questions raised by online information to your surgical team rather than acting on it independently.

CLOSING NOTE ON EVIDENCE AND INDIVIDUAL CARE

It is worth closing this appendix, and this book, with an acknowledgment of an important tension in medical care: evidence is generated from populations, but care is delivered to individuals. The statistics presented throughout this book, the percentages, the risk figures, the outcome rates, all describe populations of patients, not any single individual's certain future.

Your surgical team's role is to apply this population-level evidence to your individual situation, using their judgment, experience, and knowledge of your specific case to translate general evidence into a specific recommendation for you. This is why the relationship between patient and surgeon, the conversations, the questions, the individualised assessment, matters so much. The evidence in this book provides the foundation for understanding your situation. Your surgical team provides the individualised application of that evidence to you.

Conclusion

A LETTER TO THE PATIENT

You started reading this book in one place, perhaps uncertain, perhaps frightened, perhaps simply wanting to understand what lay ahead. I hope you are finishing it in a meaningfully different place.

Not necessarily free of anxiety, because that would be an unrealistic promise. But informed. Oriented. In possession of the knowledge you need to face what comes next with your eyes open and your questions answered.

You know what your spine is and how it works. You understand what scoliosis is, why curves progress, and what the evidence says about the long-term consequences of untreated significant scoliosis. You understand why surgery may be the right path for your situation and what the alternative trajectories look like. You know what the operation involves at a level of detail sufficient to remove the fear of the unknown. You understand the different surgical approaches, what the implants are and what they do, how anaesthesia works, and what to expect from the recovery room through the hospital stay and into the weeks and months at home. You know the risks, presented honestly, alongside the interventions and protocols in place to manage them. You know what rehabilitation requires and what it can achieve. You know what the long-term outcome data show for patients like you. And you know what to watch for, when to call your team, and what is within your control that will meaningfully influence how well you do.

That knowledge is not a small thing. Informed patients navigate this process better than uninformed ones. Not because information changes the biology of bone healing. But because it changes the patient's relationship with their own recovery. When you understand why your back hurts in a particular way at a particular stage of recovery, you are not frightened by it. When you understand why walking matters even when you would rather rest, you do it. When you understand that the emotional dip at week three is normal and temporary, you move through it rather than interpreting it as evidence that something has gone wrong.

Scoliosis surgery is a serious undertaking. I have never pretended otherwise, in these pages or in the consultation room. It asks a great deal: the courage of the decision, the preparation of the weeks before, the vulnerability of the operation itself, the patience of the months of recovery. All of this is real and should not be minimised.

But this is also real: scoliosis surgery, performed by experienced surgeons at specialist centres with dedicated teams, routinely transforms lives. Not in a single dramatic moment but in the accumulated daily reality of living without constant pain, of standing differently in the world, of wearing what you want and doing what you want and going where you want without the constant negotiation with a spine that was limiting you. The evidence I have presented in this book documents this transformation across thousands of patients followed for decades. It is not anecdote. It is data. I think about a patient I operated on years ago, a young woman who had lived with a large thoracic curve since early adolescence and who told me in our consultation that she had not worn a swimming costume in seven years, that her scoliosis was present in every social interaction she had, an invisible companion shaping every decision about clothing and activity and proximity to others. At her one-year follow-up she showed me photographs from a beach holiday where she had swum in the sea every single day. Not once. Every day.

That is what this surgery is for. Not the Cobb angle number. Not the radiographic correction percentage. The person living in the body, fully and without the constant diminishment of a condition that had been defining the edges of their life.

Your story is not finished. It is in the middle of an important chapter. And if this book has done its job, you are better equipped to navigate that chapter toward the life you deserve.

I wish you a smooth surgery, a steady recovery, and a future that surprises you with what you are capable of.

www.ingramcontent.com/pod-product-compliance
Lightning Source LLC
LaVergne TN
LVHW050814061126
851857LV00012B/794
* 9 7 9 8 2 5 6 1 7 1 9 1 9 *